INTEGRATED NUTRIENT SUPPLY MANAGEMENT SYSTEM

About the Editor

Dr. N.P. Singh (*b.* 1957) completed his M.Sc. and Ph.D. in agronomy from the Institute of Agricultural Sciences, Banaras Hindu University, Varanasi-221005 in years 1980 and 1984 respectively. He has maintained good academic record throughout his studies and recipient of District Merit Fellowship, BHU Fellowship and Pesticides India Ltd. He has joined in 1984 as a lecturer in the Department of Agronomy, College of Agriculture, North-Eastern Hill University, Medziphema, Nagaland and in 1988 he became a Reader & Head in Department of Agronomy, School of Agril. Science & Rural Development, North-Eastern Hill University, Medziphema, Nagaland. After the establishment of Nagaland University (A Central University) he was on deputation to Nagaland University up to 1996 and he joined later on as a Professor & Head, Department of Agronomy, School of Agricultural Science & Rural Development, Nagaland University, Medziphema, Nagaland.

He is a life member of different academic societies in India and abroad. In his fifteen years of teaching experience, he taught different courses in crop production and published 38 research papers, 70 popular and research articles and attended 76 conferences at regional, national and international levels. He has visited to The Netherlands, France, Thailand, and Indonesia for different academic programmes. Presently, he is working as a Principal Scientist & Head, Division of Agronomy, ICAR Research Complex for NEH Region, Umiam, Meghalaya-793103, India.

INTEGRATED NUTRIENT SUPPLY MANAGEMENT SYSTEM

(Proceeding of Seminar on Integrated Plant Nutrient Supply System on the North East Hill Region held at Medziphema)

Prof. N.P. SINGH
Department of Agronomy
School of Agricultural Science & Rural Development
Nagaland University, Medziphema-797106, Nagaland (INDIA)

CONCEPT PUBLISHING COMPANY, NEW DELHI-110059

ISBN 81-7022-977-4

First Published 2002

Published and Printed by
Ashok Kumar Mittal
Concept Publishing Company
A/15-16, Commercial Block, Mohan Garden
NEW DELHI-110059 (India)

Phones : 5648039, 5649024
Fax : 091-11-5648053
Email: publishing@conceptpub.com

FOREWORD

Fertiliser has played a key role in making our country self-sufficient in food grain production. Of the present 190 plus million tonnes of food grain production in India today, fertiliser accounts for 50 per cent of the total production as reported by FAO. Presently we had a surplus of 1 million tonnes of wheat, rice and sugar each that can be exported for valuable foreign exchange. This could not have been possible without harnessing the potential of fertiliser in raising the agriculture productivity. Accordingly, for a country like India and with fast growing population, fertiliser obviously is too important to ignore. Agriculture in the country is primarily in the hands of either illiterate or neo-literate farmers who needs to be constantly kept briefed about the modern techniques of crop husbandry. There already exists a huge gap in transferring the location specific technology to the farmers. This calls for an urgent and specified attention to all those who are connected with development of agriculture in general.

If we look at the use of fertilisers in the north-eastern hill region, it is the lowest in the country. The reasons for this are many and it is difficult to pinpoint any one of them with authority. In recent years, we have seen that the scientific use of nitrogen, phosphorus and potash has gone tremendously out of proportions. During 1994-95 the figure for the same stands at 57.7 : 26.7 : 1.0 as against the scientific ratio of 4 : 2 : 1. This is a point of serious concern for all of us to think to improve the same. It is true that shortage of phosphate and potassic fertilisers in August, 1992 leads to decline in consumption of both the fertiliser materials. If we continue to use fertilisers in the proportion we use now, our productivity will be seriously affected, so also the soil health.

Rice is the principal crop which is cultivated both in the plains and in the hills. More alternatives has to be given to raise the productivity of vegetables and fruits also. Our attention needs to be directed towards reducing the areas under shifting cultivation. We are very much committed to the agricultural development but not at the cost of soil health and our farming community. The food security so much advocated now-a-days would be impossible without the use of fertiliser in particular and other inputs in general. It hardly needs more emphasis that the growing population can be fed only by a highly fertile and production soil.

I am pleased that the Department of Agronomy, School of Agricultural Sciences and Rural Development, Nagaland University, Medziphema, Nagaland has taken initiative to organised a seminar on "Integrated Plant Nutrient Supply Management System" participated by more than hundred delegates comprising students, teachers, researchers, managers of fertiliser industries, officers and extension workers of department of Agriculture and allied departments, Government officers and farmers. The compilation of the seminar proceeding will have a document for the planners, researchers, students and progressive farmers of the region. I hope that students, researchers, planners, officers of departments of agriculture and allied departments will be benefited by this publication.

Nagaland University
HQ: Lumami, Camp Kohima
30th June, 1999

PROF. I. YANGAR
Vice-Chancellor

PREFACE

The North-Eastern Hill region of India consists of Arunachal Pradesh, Manipur, Meghalaya, Mizoram, Nagaland, Sikkim and Tripura characterised by the predominance of hilly area with considerable amount of natural resources in the shape of landmass, forestry plantations, wild life, water resources and inherent biodiversity offering considerable opportunities for holistic and integrated development of agriculture and allied sectors in a sustainable manner. The NEH region offers a great scope for growing a variety of agricultural and horticultural crops. Agriculture production in the region is mostly consumption-oriented to meet the needs of the farmers. Use of local varieties, low consumption of fertiliser and pesticides, low moisture retention capacity of upland soil, undulating difficult terrain with varying altitudes and slopes, low temperatures, no drainage in valley land during monsoon and low sunshine hours, lack of irrigation facilities during winter months, along with traditional management practices have resulted into low productivity and low cropping intensity.

Shifting cultivation is still practiced by the farmers in the region. In most of the areas only one crop of rice or maize is grown in a year during kharif season. Problem of high rainfall, soil acidity, aluminium toxicity in upland and iron toxicity in valley land have added to the problem of low agricultural productivity in this region.

This region is now passing through a crucial period with high density of population and hence increased food production is of vital importance. The food grain production in the north east hill region is not keeping pace with the rapid growth in population while the production of food grain was showing a declining trend at an annual rate of 2.18 per cent, the population in the region was growing faster at the rate of 2.43 per cent. To meet the projected food demands of the region per hectare will have to be increased by 55 per cent in 2001, nearly 100 per cent by 2010 and 190 per cent by 2025 taking the 1993-94 as the base. The region would continue to remain dependent on agriculture for many years to come as there is negligible industrial base and tourism potential had not been exploited.

No country in the world can increase the food grain production without the use of balanced doses of required nutrients. In the region low purchasing power of the farmers are the major constraints in increasing fertiliser use. Therefore, the urgent need is to increase the productivity efficiency of applied fertilisers through the use of all sources of plant nutrients like N, P and K, FYM, compost and biofertiliser which will also emerge the concept of integrated plant nutrient supply systems (IPNS). The concept of IPNS use is not fully understood by the farmers and sometimes even by extension workers. Farmers need to be made aware about the deficiencies which are coming up in soils and their effect on crop and sustainability of crop production. Soil test is one of the effective tools in obtaining balanced fertiliser recommendation. It will also help delineating nutrient deficiency area. In integrated plant nutrient supply systems, application of FYM/compost along with N-P-K fertilisers and biofertiliser the better method of supplying different plant nutrients.

Considering this, the Nagaland University, Department of Agronomy organised a Regional Seminar on "Integrated Plant Nutrient Supply Management System" to formulate and identify priority R&D programme for the NEH region. The seminar was planned and organised to share the knowledge based information and experiences generated by various R&D and other institutions over the years on a common platform for developing a IPNS strategies for the region. The seminar was addressed by officials, researchers and teachers from various States and Central Government Agencies, Universities, ICAR, Fertiliser Industries working in the North-Eastern Region and other parts of the country. The delegates participated and discussed their experiences. A good number of selected papers were contributed on the various topics related to the theme.

On behalf of the Department of Agronomy, School of Agricultural Sciences & Rural Development, Nagaland University, Medziphema, Nagaland, I extend my thanks to all the participants and those who provided direct and indirect support to make the seminar a grand success. I also thank all the contributors for sending their articles in time and sharing their data and rich experiences for the benefit of the region. The printing of the seminar proceeding has been possible due to generous support received by Nagaland University and North-Eastern Council (NEC) for which I extend my sincere thanks to the functionaries of both these institutions. I hope that papers compiled in the form of publication will go a long way to help in agricultural growth of north-eastern hill region of the country.

Medziphema, Nagaland — Prof. N.P. SINGH

WELCOME ADDRESS

Hon'ble Minister, Public Health Engineering, Shri Tokheho, Hon'ble Minister of State, Wasteland Development, Shri Rokonicha, distinguished guests, officers of the State Government of Nagaland and other North-Eastern States and Nagaland University.

Ladies and Gentlemen,

I have great pleasure in welcoming you all to this seminar organised by the Fertiliser Association of India, Eastern Region (FAI-ER) and the Department of Agronomy, Nagaland University.

At the outset, I would like to express my deep gratitude to the Hon'ble Ministers who have taken keen interest in this subject and spared their valuable time to be with us today to attend the programme. The Hon'ble Chief Minister, Shri S.C. Jamir, could not remain present today due to a pressing engagement at Delhi.

I am thankful to the Department of Agronomy for taking initiative in organising this programme and I am sure it would not have been possible without the untiring efforts made by Dr. N.P. Singh of the Department of Agronomy. He kept the key persons of the fertiliser industry as well as FAI in constant touch to join the seminar. Unfortunately, some of the very important persons of the fertiliser industry and FAI could not attend this programme due to their pre-occupation elsewhere.

To speak a few words about Nagaland, I would like to say that the fertiliser consumption in this state during 1996-97 was 3.8 kg/ha and during 1997-98 it had dropped to 2.6 kg/ha. The reasons are of course varied but it is not a healthy sign to bring about an improvement in agricultural production. Unless the fertiliser consumption is increased, the farmers of this state will not get their desired production which might dissuade them in continuing the agricultural practice in future.

I am sure the deliberation which would be made by eminent scientists and experts in this seminar would yield definite conclusions and recommendations to form a message to the farming community.

With these words, I would once again welcome you all on behalf of the FAI-ER and on my personal behalf.

Thanking you all,

S. BENERJEE
Regional Executive
The Fertiliser Association of India, Eastern Region, Calcutta

ADDRESS BY SHRI TOKHEHO YEPTHOMI MINISTER, P.H.E.

Chairman, participants of the Seminar and friends,

It gives me immense pleasure to be here with you on the occasion of the inaugural function of the Regional Seminar on "Integrated Nutrient Supply Management System with special reference to the North East Hill Region".

At the outset, I congratulate the Department of Agronomy, Nagaland University and The Fertiliser Association of India—Eastern Region, for organising this seminar on the extremely important need of proper nutrient management. I am also happy to learn that the participants of this Seminar include the Heads of Departments of Agriculture of all North-Eastern State, as also Extension personnel of Agri-Allied Departments, along with Academicians and Scientists from ICAR, SASRD, and the Agricultural Universities. I am confident that your joint consultations and efforts to find scientific solutions to the problems of agriculture in the region will go a long way in uplifting this remote and backward area of the country.

My scientific knowledge on Agricultural matters is limited, however, from a layman's point of view, I understand that management of nutrients is a must not only for increasing the yield but also for maintaining the soil fertility for sustained agricultural production. The basis of Integrated Nutrient Supply Programme (INSP) is that plant nutrients can be supplied from factory produced inorganic fertilisers and naturally occurring and locally available bulky organic manure or crop residues. Scientists and Agriculturists know that nitrogen can be supplied by simultaneous cultivation of legumes and pulses with the main crop. What is needed today, is that this knowledge available in the Agricultural Universities, must be transferred to the farmers, so that they can have a higher yield as well as preserve the soil fertility through cheaper and environment friendly means. Such as by way of a balanced use of chemical fertilisers, organic manure, green manure and bio-fertilisers like *rhizobium* and crop residue. This can be done through a coordinated effort of the scientists, officials of the Agriculture and Allied Departments and the extension workers.

The North-Eastern region constitutes seven per cent of the total land area of the country and is dominated by hilly tract. The region overwhelming comprises of difficult terrain and forests. These are probably the basic reasons why modern agriculture has not taken rapid strides. The farmers are by and large poor and either illiterate or neo-literate but they are very hard-working and the land they till is fertile. The region receives ample rainfall, and most of the arable land is rainfed. In many parts of the region Jhuming is practiced, which does not require the use of any chemical fertilisers. However, the yield in Jhum remains low and with the increasing population, pressure on Jhum lands has increased greatly. Somehow, our agricultural universities have not been able to conduct ample research in how to increase the yield in Jhum to make it economically and environmentally viable.

Lately, there has been some developments in this regard and I am happy to note that scientists have developed new interest in Jhuming. Apart from this, farmers of the north east will have to be made aware about the modern techniques of farming in order to have a green revolution in this part of the country. This is a must, in order to be able to feed the ever-increasing population. There is a need to develop technologies and techniques that are suited to the specific requirements of the region. Agricultural Scientists need to have a proper understanding of the prevalent agricultural practices in the region. Many a time, scientists, the world over, have recognised traditional knowledge and wisdom, while evolving new technologies and practices. All this can be done through an efficient mechanism of backward and forward linkages between the Scientists and the Farmers.

The fertiliser use in the region is among the lowest in the country. Due to lack of research for augmenting agricultural production in the region, the farmer is unaware of the kinds of fertilisers that are suited for his farm. This also denies the farmers of the region from taking advantage of the subsidy that is given by the Government of India on agriculture. Due to lack of awareness, farmers are also unaware of the proper mix of nitrogen, phosphate and potash that should be used. Improper use directly affects the soil fertility and hence the yield. The importance of organic fertilisers and biofertilisers need to be explained to the farmers, as they are environment friendly as well as being effective in supplying nutrients to the soil. For introducing new techniques, farmers need to be provided with both technological as well as financial support to help them adopt new technologies, and be able to meet the cost of new fertilisers and improved high yielding seeds.

In all such extension efforts the North East has an advantage over other parts of the country as our literacy rate has grown tremendously in the last two decades and we are far above the national average. The scientists, the government departments and the extension workers must keep this very important potential in mind as you plan and work towards sustaining an agricultural economy for the people of the region.

This seminar gives an opportunity for all of us to dwell on all these points and I am sure, with the presence of so many experts, scientists, officials, and field workers, many more ideas will be forthcoming on how to make the agriculture in the region, more viable. I, for one would, therefore, like to emphasise that you also have an equal responsibility in making our farmers more knowledgeable and to deliver the inputs within the easy reach of the farmers at the prices fixed by the government. I sincerely hope that you will make an honest endeavour to fulfil the need and the demand of the farmers of the region.

Before I conclude, I assure the audience that we are very much committed to agricultural development, but not at the cost of soil health and our farming community. The food security, so much advocated today would be impossible without maintaining soil fertility and productivity for which major thrust has to be given towards integrated nutrient management in achieving the goal. There is no other way that we can think to meet the food requirement not only for today, but also for the generations to come.

With these words, I take great pleasure in inaugurating the seminar on "Integrated Nutrient Supply Management System". I have firm belief that deliberations in the present seminar would help evolve constructive suggestions and recommendations, specific to the farming community of the region which will help in improvement of production by adopting Integrated Nutrient Management Technology. This is the need of the hour and in the coming millennium it will be a milestone for the economic upliftment of the farmers of the region.

Thank you,

TOKHEHO YEPTHOMI
Hon'ble PHE Minister
Government of Nagaland

VOTE OF THANKS

Hon'ble PHE Minister, Mr. Tokheho, Govt. of Nagaland, Shri Rokonicha, Minister of State, Department of Wasteland Development and Local Self-Govt., Shri T.N. Mannen, Development Commissioner & Secretary, Govt. of Nagaland, Prof. V.B. Singh, Dean & Chairman of Organising Committee, Mr. S. Benerjee, Regional Executive, The Fertiliser Association of India Eastern Region, Calcutta, Resource Persons, Guests invities, distinguished participants, Dear students, ladies and gentlemen,

At the conclusion of the inaugural function of the Regional seminar on 'Integrated Nutrient Supply Management System it is my pleasant duty to extend our gratitude to all of you for your presence here this morning.

We are deeply indebted to the Hon'ble PHE Minister Shri Tokheho for inaugurating the seminar and addressing the august gathering. Sir, you have honoured us by your esteemed presence in spite of your pre-occupation. We are indeed forth note to have you with us.

We are previleged to have Shri Rokonicha, Hon'ble Minister of State, deptt. of wasteland development and local self-government His presence on this occasion show his keen interest in agricultural development in the State as well as in the region.

We are grateful to Shri T.N. Mannen, Development Commissioner, Govt. of Nagaland for chairing the inaugural session and delivering a fruitful speech to the participants.

We express our sincere thanks to our Vice-Chancellor, Prof. I. Yangei Ao and Registrar Mr. K.K. Zhimomi for their help and encouragement for organising the regional seminar.

We express our profound gratitude to our Dean & Chairman organising committee Prof. V.B. Singh for his help and guidance to make this programme grand success.

We are also thankful to Manager of fertiliser industries, Mr. Banerjee and Mr. Ghosh from FAI, ER, Directors of various Deptts., Officers of Deptt. of Agriculture and Allied Deptts. and resource persons who are here with us today.

We are grateful to press peoples, Prashar Bharati (AIR), Doordarshan and other representative of the media for the coverage and seek their continued support.

We are extremely thankful to commandent of 27 AR, 45 BN CRPF, 1st NAP, Project Director, NRC for Mithum, Joint Director, ICAR Research Complex for their help to organise the seminar and I hope that in future they provide the support.

We wish to express our sincere thanks to all the staff of school, Govt. officer of Medziphema, G.B. of Medziphema village and town, chairmen of village council and town committee, president of youth organisation and elderly people of Medziphema village and town.

We express our thanks to the students, who are the driving force for arrangement of auditorium and various materials arrangement connected with regional seminar.

On behalf of the organising committee and my own behalf, I express my sincere thanks to each and everyone those who help us directly and indirectly to make this programme a grand success.

May I thank you all once again and invite you to join us for a cup of coffee outside the auditorium.

Thanking you,

Prof. N.P. SINGH
Organising Secretary
Deptt. of Agronomy
NU, SASARD, Medziphema, Nagaland

FERTILISER PRICE AND SUBSIDY

The fertiliser consumption pattern of N, P_2O_5 and K_2O, if observed over the last 10 years indicates a drop in the consumption of P_2O_5 and K_2O from 1992-93. A significant policy change was adopted by the Government of India (GOI) in August '92 wherein the pricing and distribution in P & K fertilisers were decontrolled. This meant that the manufacturers and suppliers were at liberty to fix the prices of these fertilisers as per the market force and could sell the fertilisers in any part of the country. This had led to tremendous rise in the prices of these fertilisers. Subsequently, the GOI introduced a scheme of adhoc concession w.e.f. 1-10-92 under which concession at prescribed rates was provided to bring down the selling prices to the farmers. The GOI provided a lump sum amount to each state to reimburse the manufacturers and suppliers the subsidy amount depending upon the sale of their materials.

Further, the State Governments were entrusted with the responsibility of fixing the prices of decontrolled fertilisers. These had led to price differences from state to state. The GOI finally took the responsibility themselves to fix uniform prices of all decontrolled fertilisers which would be applicable for all the states in the country. Further, GOI decided that the subsidy reimbursement would be made by them based on the verified bills of sale made by the manufacturers/suppliers in each state. Presently, this practice is invoke and the manufacturer and supplier get their subsidy reimbursement directly from the GOI after their bills of sale are duly certified by the State Government where the sale is made.

The present maximum retail price (exclusive of sales tax and other taxes) and the subsidy amount for each fertiliser is indicated in the table.

Any materials sold by any manufacturer/supplier at the MRP or below the MRP would be eligible for the subsidy indicated against each MRP. It may be mentioned here that only in case of SSP, the GOI has given the responsibility to the respective State Government to fix the MRP for both powder and granuler and the subsidy reimbursible per

(*Rs./tonne*)

	MRP	Adhoc Cession
DAP—Indigenous	8,300	4,400
DAP—Imported	8,300	3,000
MOP	3,700	3,000
10 : 26 : 26	7,300	3,777
12 : 32 : 16	7,400	3,827
14 : 28 : 14	7, 300	3,590
14 : 35 : 14	7,500	4,071
15 : 15 : 15	6,200	2,814
16 : 20 : 0	6,400	2,477
17 : 17 : 17	7,200	3,189
19 : 19 : 19	7,300	3,564
20 : 20 : 0	6,500	2,752
23 : 23 : 0	7,100	3,165
28 : 28 : 0	8,000	3,853

tonne of SSP sold is Rs. 900/tonne. Each State Government before the onset of season, i.e. *Kharif* and *Rabi* fixes the price of SSP for their state.

S. BANERJEE

LIST OF CONTRIBUTORS

Anand, S.S., Jt. General Manager (M), IFFCO, 8 Acharya J.C. Bose Road, Circular Court, Calcutta-17 (W.B.).

Ayemi, S. Yehoto, Director, Department of Agriculture, Govt. of Nagaland, Kohima, Nagaland.

Bhattacharyya, H.C., Agronomist, Regional Crop Research Station, Assam Agricultural University, Titabar, Assam.

Bhave, V.J., Deputy General Manager, Rastriya Chemicals and Fertiliser Ltd., 'Priyadarshini Eastern Highway Express, Mumbai-400022, Maharashtra.

Biswas, B.C., Chief Agronomist, The Fertiliser Association of India, 10, Shaheed Jit Singh Marg, New Delhi-110067.

Chetri, Dipak, Dy. Director (Fertiliser) Department of Agriculture, Government of Nagaland, Kohima, Nagaland.

Chuba AO, K., Director, Department of Horticulture, Government of Nagaland, Kohima, Nagaland.

(Mrs.) Deka, Medhi B., Agricultural Chemist, Agricultural Chemistry Research Unit, Assam Agricultural University, Jorhat-785013, Assam.

Gupta, R.C., Head, Deptt. of Soil Science and Agril. Chemistry, School of Agril. Sciences and Rural Development, Nagaland University, Medziphema-797106, Nagaland.

Joshi, L., General Manager (Marketing) Pyrites, Phosphates and Chemical Ltd. (A Govt. of India Undertaking), Noida-201301 (UP).

Kar, A.K., Hindustan Lever Chemical Ltd., Illaco House, 1&3 Brabourne Road, Calcutta-1 (W.B.).

Kar, P.L., Visiting Professor, Department of Horticulture, Nagaland University, School of Agril. Sciences and Rural Development, Medziphema-797106, Nagaland.

Medhi, D.N., Associate Professor, Deptt. of Agronomy, Assam Agricultural University, Jorhat-785013, Assam.

Roychoudhury, S., Asstt. Microbiologist, Regional Biofertiliser Development Centre, CAU Campus, Iroisemba, Imphal, Manipur.

Saha, S.K., Manager (Agricultural Services) Pyrites, Phosphates and Chemicals Ltd. (A Govt. of India undertaking), Noida-201301 (UP).

Sharma, A.C., Department of Agronomy, Assam Agricultural University, Jorhat-785013, Assam.

Singh, N.P., Head, Department of Agronomy, School of Agril. Sciences and Rural Development, Nagaland University, Medziphema-797106, Nagaland.

Singh, V.B., Dean, Nagaland University, School of Agricultural Sciences and Rural Development, Medziphema-797106, Nagaland.

Upadhayay, D.N., Head, Department of Plant Pathology, School of Agricultural Sciences and Rural Development, Nagaland University, Medziphema-797106, Nagaland.

Yadav, A.K., Regional Director, Regional Biofertiliser Development Centre, CAU Campus, Iroisemba, Imphal, Manipur.

CONTENTS

LIST OF TABLES

LIST OF FIGURES

1

FERTILISER PRODUCTION, MARKETING AND USE IN INDIA WITH REFERENCE TO EAST AND NORTH-EASTERN REGION

— *B.C. Biswas*

ABSTRACT

India has emerged as the third producer and consumer of fertiliser in the world after the fall of USSR. Fertiliser use in India is imbalanced regionally and nutritionality. It has become more imbalance after the decontrol of P & K fertiliser in August 1992 and consequent price hike. The paper deals with fertiliser production, marketing and use in India with reference to East and North-Eastern region.

Introduction

Fertiliser industry is as old as agricultural research in the country. Fertiliser production (SSP) started in Ranipet in Tamil Nadu in 1906 while Imperial Agriculture Research Institute (IARI) started in 1905 in old Pusa, Bihar. In first 40 years of the present century fertiliser production and consumption were very low, practically nil in case of foodgrains. During 1942-43, India witnessed a tragic famine known as Bengal famine which took away the lives of millions. To boost up foodgrains production, "Grow More Food Campaign" having fertiliser as the key component, was launched. The first public fertiliser unit was set up at Sindri, Bihar in 1951.

The next 15 years infrastructural facilities for soil fertility evaluation, irrigation and HYV seed production etc. were developed. Real thrust in foodgrain production came in mid-60s with introduction of HYV seeds of wheat, rice and other cereals which demanded high amount of fertiliser for their proper expression of yield potential. Fertiliser production and consumption also expanded very rapidly from mid-60s to cope up with the demand.

India now occupies the third position in production and consumption of fertiliser in the World. However, there exist, nutrient-wise and regional imbalances in fertiliser consumption. In East and North-Eastern region having its own problem, consumes less amount of fertiliser in foodgrain production. This paper deals with the production, marketing and consumption of fertiliser in India with reference to East and North-Eastern States.

Production and Product Pattern

The favourable Government policies and pragmatic approaches towards the administrative action in the past resulted in rapid growth of installed capacity in private, cooperative and public sectors. India produces only N and P fertilisers and entire potash (K) requirement is made through imports because India has no K mine in the country. The installed capacity of N & P increased from 0.35 mt. in 1960-61 to 12.14 mt. in 1994-95 (Table 1.1) and the total production of these two fertilisers reached a landmark of 10 mt. during 1994-95.

Table 1.1: Capacity of N and P Nutrients

(Million MT)

Year	N	P_2O_5
1950-51	0.017	0.021
1960-61	0.246	0.107
1970-71	1.515	0.532
1980-81	4.736	1.386
1990-91	8.211	2.771
1994-95	9.193	2.943

Production includes a whole range of N & P fertiliser (Table 1.2). It is interesting to note that there has been a remarkable shift from low analysis to high analysis fertilisers (HAF) product over the years because of lower cost of transport of HAF. During 1994-95 urea accounted for 82 per cent of total N fertiliser production in the country while DAP is the most dominating source of P fertiliser having the contribution of about 51 per cent P_2O_5 production (Table 1.3).

Sector-wise capacity and production are given in Table 1.4 which indicate that with 47.4 per cent share in N capacity, public sector plants contribute 36.8 per cent of production. The N capacity utilisation (67.2%) of public sector units is much lower than those of private (109.4%) and cooperative (109.8%) sector. In P, private sector accounts for 61.3 per cent of P_2O_5 capacity with production share of 58.2 per cent while cooperative sector with 10.9 per cent share in capacity contributed for 14.8 per cent of P_2O_5 production and also achieved the highest capacity utilisation of 122.3 per cent in 1994-95.

Table 1.2: Capacity and Production of Fertiliser Products and Intermediates (1994-95)

(Million MT)

Intermediate/Product	Capacity	Production
Ammonia	11.33	9.26
Sulphuric Acid	6.75	3.94*
Phosphoric Acid	0.73	0.43
Urea	16.65	14.14
Ammonium Chloride (ACl)	0.13	0.14
Ammonium Sulphate (AS)	1.09	0.58
Calcium Ammonium Nitrate (CAN)	0.94	0.57
Single Super Phosphate (SSP)	5.27	3.02
Diammonium Phosphate (DAP)	2.31	2.82
Complex Fertilisers (NP/NPKs)	3.69	3.59

* Data for 1991-92.

Table 1.3: Share of Products in Fertiliser Production (1994-95)

Product	% Share of Total Nutrient	
	N	P
Urea	81.9	—
Other N Fertilisers	3.7	—
DAP	6.4	50.7
SSP	—	18.9
Other NP/NPK	8.0	30.4
	100.0	100.0

Table 1.4: Statewise Share of Capacity and Production of N and P_2O_5 Capacity Utilisation (1994-95)

(Per cent)

Sector	Share of Capacity		Share of Production		Capacity Utilisation	
	N	P_2O_5	N	P_2O_5	N	P_2O_5
Public	47.4	27.9	36.8	27.0	67.2	87.5
Cooperative	16.7	10.9	21.2	14.8	109.8	122.3
Private	35.9	61.3	42.0	58.2	109.4	88.4
Total	100.0	100.0	100.0	100.0	88.9	91.9

Feedstock

Though India uses various feedstocks for fertiliser production, of late, natural gas has emerged the predominant feedstock in production of ammonia and nitrogenous fertilisers in the country. Naphtha and fuel oil occupy the second and third position respectively (Table 1.5) on feedstocks for ammonia production. A list of ammonia plants with their capacity, feedstock and year of commissioning is indicated in Table 1.6.

Table 1.5: Feedstockwise Share in Total Capacity and Production with Capacity Utilisation of N (1994-95)

(Per cent)

Feedstock	Capacity	Production	Capacity Utilisation
Natural/Associated gas	47.7	49.5	95.3
Naphtha	27.4	26.1	82.6
Fuel Oil	13.6	15.0	95.3
Coal	5.0	0.8	14.4
COG	0.7	0.5	61.3
External Ammonia	5.0	7.2	126.3
Others	0.7	0.7	94.7
Total	100.0	100.0	88.9

Table 1.6: List of Ammonia Plants Unit Capacity and Feedstock

	Year of Commissioning	Capacity in TPD	Employed Feedstock	Type of Compressor
(1)	(2)	(3)	(4)	(5)
I. Before 1970				
1. FACT Alwaye	1960	355	Nap.	RC
1a. NFL Nangal	1961/89	300	Electrolysis/Nap	RC
2. RCF Trombay-I	1965	350	N.G.	RC
3. NLC Neyveli	1966/79	285	Lignite/F.O.	RC
4. CLF Visakhapatnam	1967	357	Nap	RC
5. GSFC Baroda-I	1967	500	N.G.	RC
GSFC Baroda-II		450	N.G.+Nap	
6. HFC Namrup-I	1969	200	N.G.	CC
HFC Namrup-II		600	N.G.	
7. Duncans Kanpur	1969	415	Nap.	CC
		830	Nap.	
8. SAIL Rourkela	1969	450	Nap.	RC

(Contd.)

Table 1.6: (*Contd.*)

(1)	(2)	(3)	(4)	(5)
9. FCI Gorakhpur	1969	550	Nap.	RC not in Oprn.
10. SFC Kota	1969	600	Nap.	RC
II. 1971-75				
1. MFL Madras	1971	750	Nap.	CC
2. FACT Cochin	1973	600	Nap.	CC
3. ZACL Goa	1973	660	Nap.	CC
4. HFC Durgapur	1974	600	Nap.	CC
5. IFFCO Kalol	1975	910	N.G.	CC
6. SPIC Tuticorin	1975	1100	Nap.	CC
III. 1976-80				
1. HFC Barauni	1976	600	Nap.	CC
2. MCFL Mangalore	1976	660	Nap.	CC
3. NFL Nangal	1978	900	F.O.	CC
4. FCI Sindri	1979	900	F.O.	CC
5. NFL Bathinda	1979	900	F.O.	CC
6. NFL Panipat	1979	900	F.O.	CC
7. FCI Ramagundam	1980	900	Coal	CC
8. FCI Talcher	1980	900	Coal	CC
IV. 1981-85				
1. IFFCO Phulpur	1981	900	Nap.	CC
2. RCF Trombay V	1982	900	N.G.	CC
3. GNFC Bharuch	1982	1350	F.O.	CC
4. RCF Thal	1985	2×1350	N.G.	CC
V. After 1985				
1. KRIBHCO Hazira	1986	2×1350	N.G.	CC
2. HFC Namrup III	1987	600	N.G.	CC
3. IGFCC Jagdishpur	1988	1350	N.G.	CC
4 IFFCO Aonla	1988	1350	N.G.	CC
5. NFL Vijaipur	1988	1350	N.G.	CC
6. DFFCL Taloja	1992	272	N.G.	CC
7. NFCL Kakinada	1992	900	N.G.	CC
8. CFCL Gadepan	1994	1350	N.G.	CC
9. TCL Babrala	1994	1350	N.G.	CC
10. Oswal Shahjahanpur	1995	1350	N.G.	CC

Notes: RC—Reciprocating Compressor
CC—Centrifugal Compressor.

Almost all ammonia plants are parts of ammonia-urea complexes. A total of 38 urea plants with a capacity of about 16.65 mt. were in operation during 1994-95. A list of the urea plants is given in Table 1.7. There are also two ammonium chloride, two ammonium sulphate and three CAN plants to produce N fertilisers. About 80 SSP plants produce about 5 mt. SSP.

Table 1.7: A List of Urea Plants—Capacity and Technology

	Capacity in TPD	Technology
I. Before 1970		
1. RCF Trombay-I	300	Chemico
2. NLC Neyveli	465	Montedison
3. CFL Visakhapatnam	400	CPI Allied
4. GSFC Baroda	1100	Mitsui-Toatsu
5. HFC Namrup-II	1000	Montedison
6. FCI Gorakhpur	950	Mitsuli-Toatsu
7. SFC Kota	1000	Stamicarbon
8. DIL Kanpur	1364 + 682	Mitsui-Toatsu
II. 1971-75		
1. MFL Madras	640	Chemico
2. FACT Cochin	1000	Montedison
3. ZACL Goa	1140	Mitsui-Toatsu
4. HFC Durgapur	1000	Montedison
5. IFFCO Kalol	1200	Stamicarbon
6. SPIC Tuticorin	1530	Mitsui-Toatsu
III. 1976-80		
1. HFC Barauni	1000	Montedison
2. MCFL Mangalore	1000	Stamicarbon
3. NFL Nangal	1000	Montedison
4 FCI Sindri	1000	Montedison
5. NFL Bathinda	1500	Montedison
6. NFL Panipat	1550	Mitsui-Toatsu
7. FCI Ramagundam	1500	Montedison
8. FCI Talcher	1500	Montedison
IV. 1981-85		
1. IFFCO Phulpur	1500	Snamprogetti
2. RCF Trombay-V	1000	Snamprogetti
3. GNFC Bharuch	1800	Snamprogetti
4. RCF Thal	3×1500	Snamprogetti
V. After 1985		
1. KRIBHCO Hazira	4×1100	Snamprogetti
2. HFC Namrup-III	1167	PDIL
3. IGFCC Jagdishpur	2×1100	Snamprogetti
4. IFFCO Aonle	2×1100	Snamprogetti
5. NFL Vijaipur	2×1100	Snamprogetti
6. NFCL Kakinada	1500	Snamprogetti
7. CFCL Gadepan	2×1100	Snamprogetti
8. TCL Babrala	2×1100	Snamprogetti
9. Oswal Shahjahanpur	2×1100	Snamprogetti

Production Efficiency and Future Strategies

Capacity utilisation of N fertiliser plants improved from 63 per cent in 1970-71 to 89 per cent in 1994-95. The improvement in P fertiliser production was from 53 to 92 per cent during the same period (Table 1.8). Average energy consumption for ammonia production also increased from 14.8 G cal/mt. ammonia in 1979-80 to 11.0 G cal/mt. in 1994-95. Similar improvement in energy consumption has also been effected in urea plants (7.91 G cal/mt. during 1994-95).

Table 1.8: Production and Capacity Utilisation of Nitrogen and Phosphatic Fertilisers

Year	Production (Million MT)		Capacity Utilisation (%)	
	N	P	N	P
1970-71	0.83	0.23	63	53
1980-81	2.16	0.84	53	65
1990-91	6.99	2.05	86	75
1994-95	7.94	2.56	89	92

Domestic production of fertilisers is not enough to meet the consumption. Therefore, the country imported 3.1 mt. of NPK during 1994-95 (Table 1.9). The likely import during 1995-96 would be about 3.6 mt. of Urea and 1.5 mt. of DAP and 100 per cent need of K.

Table 1.9: Average Energy Consumption of Ammonia Production in India

Year	Capacity Utilisation (%)	Energy Consumption (G.Cal/MT)
1979-80	63	14.8
1985-86	72	13.7
1987-88	76	12.5
1993-94	85	11.5
1994-95	88	11.0

This indicates the need of expansion of production capacity further. But there are serious constraints of feedstock. Our new capacities are mainly gas based. But availability of gas is becoming constraint. Naphtha is, therefore, the choice for feedstock for ammonia and urea plants. But its availability in India is also a problem, so it has to be imported at international prices.

The plants commissioned in mid-60s and early 70s, particularly ones in PS suffer from design efficiencies and equipment problem.

Their rehabilitation is urgently required. Very old plant of course, need complete replacement. Gas based, new generation plants are very efficient. But still there is scope of improvement. Adequate investment on revamping of existing plants will add production and efficiency both.

In case of P, India's condition is not satisfactory, because it has to depend heavily on raw material, namely rock phosphate and sulphur and intermediates (phosphoric acid), DAP import, therefore, would continue. Of course, strategy should be to produce the fertiliser material in India based on imported raw material and phos-acid. The joint venture abroad for production of phos-acid may help to reduce our dependence on phos-acid. Our phos-acid capacity also should be increased.

Though urea and DAP would continue to dominate India's production scene in future, there is a need to diversify the fertiliser production. The thrust area are to produce fertiliser to increase use efficiency and quality. It has become more important after the decontrol of P & K fertilisers.

Fertiliser Consumption and Marketing

Use of fertiliser began in India at the close of the last century with the fertilisation of tea and coffee plantation. The use of fertiliser in foodgrains started slowly picking up in the 40s with the free distribution of ammonium sulphate to farmers under the "Grow More Food Campaign".

Although fertiliser consumption increased gradually over the next quarter of the century, the growth rate was not spectacular. For example the consumption went up from 66,000 tonnes in 1951-52 to 785 thousand tonnes during 1965-66. The consumption per ha of cropped area increased from 0.5 kg. to 5.05 kg. during the same period.

Marketing in the accepted sense hardly existed in the case of fertiliser in India till mid-60s. The emphasis was more on distribution with only limited emphasis in a few area of market development and promotion. Scientific and aggressive marketing of fertiliser really started with implementation of recommendation of Sivaraman Committee (1965) and the setting up of large new capacity in country coinciding with the introduction of HYV seeds of foodgrains.

It was realised that food production in the country could be increased by using ever-increasing quantities of chemical fertilisers. It was also recognised that domestic manufacturers had an important role to play in this regard. Other factors were the increase in irrigated area, intensive agricultural research efforts to evoke new farming technology suited for the new varieties of crops under different agroclimatic conditions and measures for rapid transfer of technology to the farmers' field.

Fertiliser consumption rose to 1.1 mt. in the year 1966-67, an increase of 40 per cent over the previous year. Consumption continued to rise every year thereafter so fast that it was more than doubled in 1970-71 compared to 1966-67. This increase represented an average compound growth rate of nearly 25 per cent per annum.

The year 1966-67 could be rightly called as the watershed that divide the earlier "epoch of fertiliser distribution" from the present era of fertiliser marketing. Today, a wider range of straight and complex grades of fertiliser are marketed through modern sophisticated and integrated marketing system and the farmer can select the material he wants to use. In the 70s, the momentum to the growth in consumption slowed down somewhat. To start with, availability was a constraint for about a year. Soon thereafter came oil crisis and consequential increase in the price of fertiliser by 100—150 per cent. Farmers would not just accept the fertiliser at that price and consumption went down in 1974-75 compared to the previous year, for the time after many years. The overall drop was 9.3 per cent.

The position was alarming. Various corrective measures like reduction of fertiliser prices, introduction of fertiliser promotional activities revived the upsurge in consumption. Consumption went up by 12.4 and 17.9 per cent in 1975-76 and 1976-77 respectively.

Retention Price Scheme (RPS) introduced after the oil crisis, had made a very favourable impact on production, marketing and use of fertiliser for the next 15 years or so. It was really a golden era of fertiliser sector.

The year 1977-78 and 1978-79 were very favourable for fertiliser consumption and growth rates of 25 per cent and 19.4 per cent were registered. The NPK consumption reached 5 mt. mark during 1977-78. Timely availability of fertilisers, higher VCR, increase area under irrigation and HYV crop, better promotional work etc. were the factors responsible for the same.

In 1979-80, the country experienced one of the worst droughts of the century. The problem was compounded by widespread shortage of power and diesel. This put heavy constraints on the agricultural front. Consumption and production of fertiliser were affected alike.

During 1980-81 fertiliser consumption increased by 5.0 per cent in spite of 38 per cent increase in price. As a result of another price like in July 1981 the consumption increase was only 7 per cent. The highlights of the next 10 years were (i) that price remained the same, (ii) in

1987-88 there was serious drought resulting in drastic reduction in fertiliser consumption and agricultural production, and (iii) but 1988-89 was very good year resulting in 25 per cent increase in fertiliser consumption and all time record foodgrain production. Fertiliser consumption was seriously affected after decontrol of P & K fertiliser in August 1992 (Table 1.10).

Table 1.10: Nutrient Consumption and Growth Rate per Annum in India 1951-52 to 1994-95

Year	Consumption ('000 tonnes)				Rate of Growth of $N + P_2O_5 + K_2O$ per annum (%)*
	N	P_2O_5	K_2O	Total	
1951-52	58.7	6.9	—	65.6	—
1960-61	211.7	53.1	29.0	293.8	17.6
1965-66	574.8	132.5	77.3	784.6	21.7
1983-84	5,204.4	1,730.3	775.4	7,710.1	20.4
1987-88	5,716.8	2,187.1	880.5	8,784.3	1.6
1988-89	7,251.0	2,720.7	1,068.4	11,040.1	25.7
1991-92	8,046.3	3,321.2	1,360.6	12,728.0	1.4
1992-93	8,426.8	2,843.8	883.9	12,154.5	-4.5
1993-94**	8,788.6	2,699.3	908.4	12,366.3	1.7
1994-95**	9,511.1	2,944.7	1,064.4	13,520.2	9.3

* Compound growth rate per annum from 1951-52 to 1988-89.
** Provisional.

Statewise nutrient consumption per unit of gross cropped area during 1992-93 to 1994-95 is shown in Table 1.11.

Table 1.12 indicates consumption of fertilisei nutrients per hectare of arable land in some selected countries during 1992-93 and 1993-94.

Table 1.11: Consumption of Plant Nutrients ($N + P_2O_5 + K_2O$) Per Unit of Gross Cropped Area, 1992-93 to 1994-95

(kg/ha)

States	Consumption ($N + P_2O_5 + K_2O$)			Ranking (1994-95)
	1992-93	1993-94@	1994-95@	
(1)	(2)	(3)	(4)	(5)
Punjab	159.5	159.5	170.9	1
Haryana	109.3	120.5	127.9	2
Andhra Pradesh	114.8	117.0	125.2	3
Tamil Nadu	114.6	111.9	113.4	4
Uttar Pradesh	84.4	88.7	96.0	5
West Bengal	84.4	86.0	86.6	6

(Contd.)

Table 1.11: (*Contd.*)

(1)	(2)	(3)	(4)	(5)
Gujarat	68.2	63.7	77.9	7
Maharashtra	56.4	59.5	69.2	8
Karnataka	63.0	65.0	67.5	9
Kerala	67.2	58.5	65.1	10
Bihar	58.7	57.7	64.3	11
Jammu & Kashmir	41.1	39.2	47.1	12
Madhya Pradesh	34.3	33.5	38.8	13
Rajasthan	27.1	27.8	33.3	14
Himachal Pradesh	31.2	29.2	29.8	15
Orissa	20.7	21.2	22.4	16
Assam	6.9	8.7	10.9	17
All-India	66.5	67.7	74.0	

@ Provisional.

Table 1.12: Consumption of Fertiliser Nutrients (N + P_2O_5 + K_2O) Per Hectare of Arable Land and Land Under Permanent Crop, 1992-93 and 1993-94

Country	Kg/hectare	
	1992-93	1993-94
Australia	27.8	31.9
Netherlands	587.5	559.9
Germany	238.7	220.5
Japan	395.1	407.1
United Kingdom	303.2	338.0
Egypt	328.1	357.0
France	235.4	237.2
Korea Rep.	465.5	473.8
Italy	160.1	147.6
China	306.0	261.4
Pakistan	101.7	101.0
Bangladesh	107.2	97.0
India	71.7	72.9
World	87.3	83.4

Economic Reforms and Fertiliser Sector

Consequent to economic reforms implemented during middle 1991 by Government of India, fertiliser sector also came under its purview. Highlights of some important policy changes are listed below:

July 1991

(i) Ammonium Sulphate, Calcium Ammonium Nitrate and

Ammonium Chloride customarily known as Low Analysis Fertilisers, were decontrolled.

(ii) The controlled selling prices of all other fertilisers were raised by 40 per cent.

(iii) A subsidy ceiling on Single Superphosphate was introduced.

August 1992—Decontrol of P & K

(i) All P & K bearing fertilisers were decontrolled.

(ii) Ammonium Sulphate, Calcium Ammonium Nitrate and Ammonium Chloride were brought back within the purview of control.

(iii) The selling price of urea which continued to be under control was reduced by 10 per cent.

September 1992—Decanalisation of DAP

In disguise of liberalisation of import policy, Government of India sprang another blow to Indian Fertiliser Industry by decanalisation of import of DAP at zero rate of duty.

October 1992—Provision of Ad hoc Subsidy

Within about a month of its policy to decontrol of P & K, Government of India realised that farmers will not be able to pay such an increase in the prices of decontrolled fertilisers. Consequently, it made a provision of Rs. 3.4 billion to be passed on to the farmers as 'ad hoc subsidy' to cushion the impact of the increase in prices of decontrolled fertilisers except SSP with the following criteria.

The highlights of the scheme were:

(i) The concessions (ad hoc subsidy) proposed to be extended to the farmer would be Rs. 1000 per tonne each for DAP and MOP and ranging from Rs. 435 to Rs. 999 per tonne for complexes.

(ii) Indicative farm gate prices of DAP and MOP were Rs. 6500 and Rs. 4200 per tonne respectively.

(iii) The scheme was applicable on sales during October-December 1992 initially and later was extended upto March 1993.

(iv) The scheme was to be implemented by State Governments.

(v) A budget provision of Rs. 2.0, 0.5 and 0.9 billion was made for DAP, complexes and MOP respectively.

May 1993—Reintroduction of Ad hoc Subsidy for 1992-93

The highlights of the scheme were:

(i) The scheme was to be implemented by State Governments;
(ii) A band of prices was indicated for Kharif 1993;
(iii) SSP was included in the scheme;
(iv) Only indigenous DAP was eligible for the ad hoc subsidy ;
(v) The scheme was operative for 1993-94;
(vi) Funds allocated for one product will not be diverted for sale of other product;
(vii) The concessions were applicable on sales from 12th June:

June 1993—Decanalisation of imported MOP, SOP and MAP.
June 1994—Continuation of Ad hoc Subsidy for 1993-94.
June 1994—Price Revision:

(1) Urea prices were increased by 20 per cent w.e.f. June 10, 1994.
(2) CAN, ACI and AS were decontrolled from price, movement and distribution.

1995-96—Continuation of Ad hoc Subsidy.

Impact of Policy Changes

While the economic reforms under a liberalised system have been implemented by the Government and is being lauded as a step towards making nation strong and economically and financially sound in the world, various sectors have been treated at par. The application of economic policies cannot be at par for various sectors and fertiliser sector has certainly paid the price as explained below:

Fertiliser Production

While the country was progressing successfully towards achieving self-sufficiency in fertiliser production, it suffered during 1992-93 and 1993-94 (Table 1.13). Our target of producing 10 million tonnes of $N + P_2O_5$ has so far eluded. The total production of N and P_2O_5 has declined after attaining a peak during 1991-92 mainly because of shortfall in the production of DAP and SSP on account of decontrol of P and K fertilisers in August 1992. After that, significant improvement on the production of Urea, DAP, SSP and Complexes (NP/NPKs) resulted in positive growth during 1994-95.

Table 1.13: Fertiliser Production during 1990-91 to 1994-95

('000 MT)

Fertiliser	Year				
	1990-91	1991-92	1992-93	1993-94	1994-95
N	6,993.1	7,301.5	7,430.6	7,231.2	7,994.3
P_2O_5	2,051.1	2,561.6	2,320.8	1,874.3	2,556.7
Total	9,044.2	9,863.1	9,751.4	9,100.9	10,551.0
Urea	12,835.9	12,831.3	13,125.9	13,150.2	14,137.1
DAP	1,904.9	2,873.6	2,598.8	1,951.5	2,820.1
SSP	3,650.3	2,984.8	2,330.9	2,257.2	3,042.6*

* Including production of SSP (14% w.s. P_2O_5).

Fertiliser Consumption

Similar decreasing trend in fertiliser consumption has also been observed during 1992-93 and 1993-94 whereas during 1993-94 there was slight improvement mainly because of spurt in urea consumption (Table 1.14).

Table 1.14: Fertiliser Consumption during 1990-91 to 1994-95

('000 MT)

Fertiliser	Year				
	1990-91	1991-92	1992-93	1993-94	1994-95
N	7,997.2	8,046.3	8,426.8	8,788.6	9.511.1
P_2O_5	3,221.0	3,321.2	2,843.8	2,669.3	2,944.7
K_2O	1,328.0	1,360.6	883.9	908.4	1,064.4
Total	12,546.2	12,728.0	12,154.5	12,366.3	13,520.2
Urea	14,073.6	14,003.3	14,905.4	15,830.4	17.067.6
DAP	4,248.1	4,517.7	4,052.0	3,480.1	3,589.6
SSP	3,558.2	3,164.8	2,008.5	2,352.6	2,656.6
MOP	1,631.0	1,700.9	974.3	1,052.5	1,188.4

Urea consumption which was stagnant during 1990-91 and 1991-92 increased by almost 900, 925 and 1240 thousand tonnes during 1992-93, 1993-94 and 1994-95 respectively. It is presumed that partial increases in the consumption of urea is on account of decrease in the consumption of DAP. After consuming about 4.5 million tonnes of DAP during 1991-92, the fall during 1992-93 and 1993-94 has been quite steady. In 1994-

95 slight improvement was noticed in DAP and SSP. The fertiliser consumption targets were finalised by National Informatic Centre (NIC) of Planning Commission, Government of India at the time of submission of Eighth Five Year Plan Document sometime during 1989. The fertiliser consumption had been steadily increasing as per the targets fixed by NIC upto 1991-92 (Fig. 1.1). It may be seen that the consumption of nitrogen has also been affected though increased consumption of urea has taken place. The actual N consumption is much below the target upto 1993-94 (Fig. 1.2). However, after the decontrol of phosphatic and

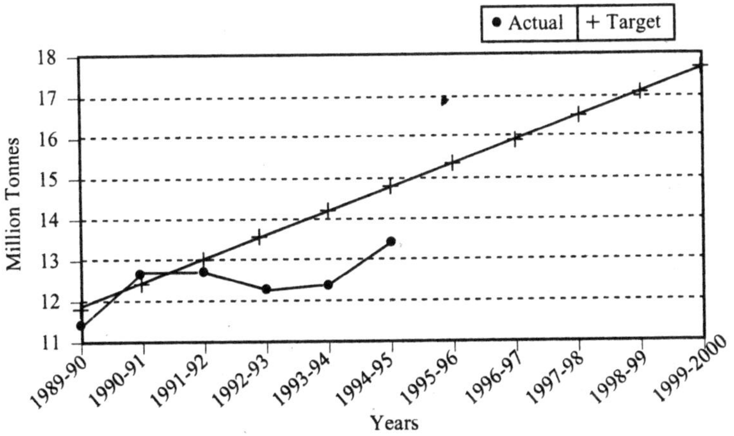

Fig. 1.1: Target and Consumption of Fertiliser ($N + P_2O_5 + K_2O$) 1989-90 to 1999-2000

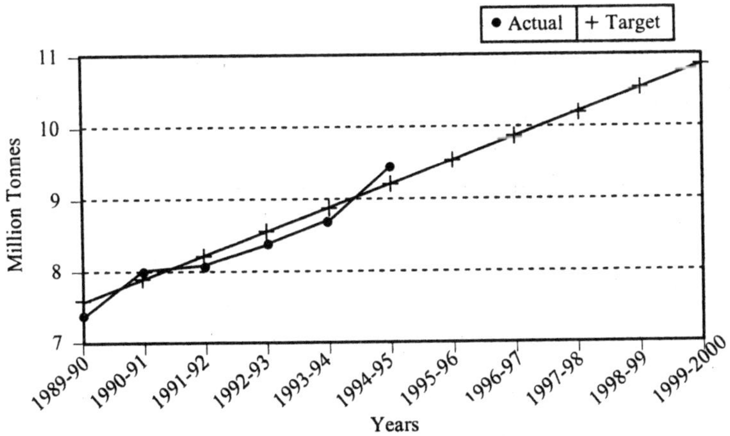

Fig. 1.2: Target and Consumption of Fertiliser—N 1989-90 to 1999-2000

potassic fertilisers, there has been a steep fall in the consumption of P_2O_5 (Fig. 1.3), K_2O (Fig. 1.4) and DAP (Fig. 1.5). The trend of decreased consumption of P_2O_5 and K_2O is to be arrested and brought back to the original targets failing which it would affects the crop yields in the long run.

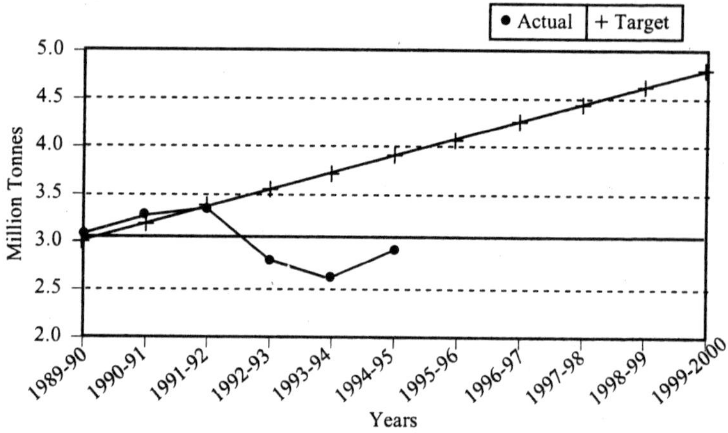

Fig. 1.3: Target and Consumption of Fertiliser—P_2O_5 1989-90 to 1999-2000

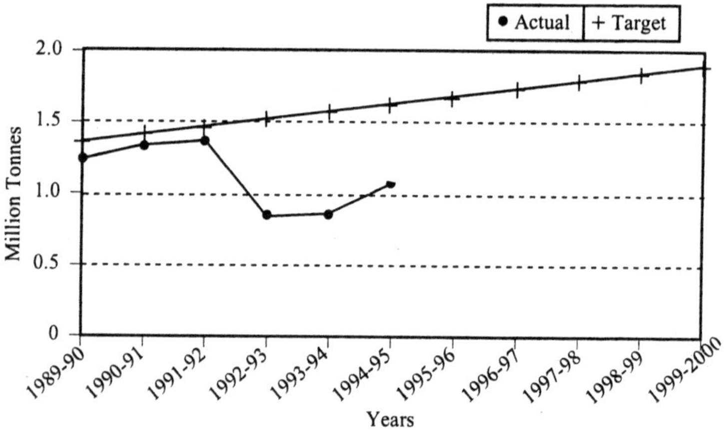

Fig. 1.4: Target and Consumption of Fertiliser—K_2O 1989-90 to 1999-2000

Fertiliser Imports

Urea and DAP is imported to bridge the gap between demand and supply whereas 100 per cent of demand of MOP is imported since no

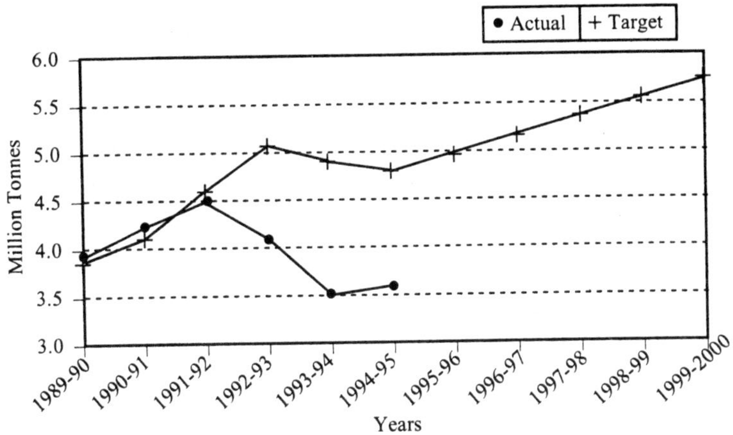

Fig. 1.5: Target and Consumption of DAP 1989-90 to 1999-2000

MOP is produced in the country. Because of uncertain atmosphere regarding the production and government policies of ad hoc concessions on DAP, the import of DAP has not been consistent with the demand (Table 1.15). While the overall consumption of DAP has reduced, the import of DAP has also reduced.

Table 1.15: Fertiliser Import during 1990-91 to 1995-96

('000 MT)

Fertiliser	Year				
	1990-91	1991-92	1992-93	1993-94	1994 95
Urea	Nil	391	1857	2840	2884
DAP	2155	2077	1533	1569	792
MOP	2120	2040	1761	1428	2120

NPK Ratio

Because of the pragmatic agriculture policies and efforts by the Scientists, the NPK ratio over a period of time has been narrowing until the Kharif 1992 (Table 1.16). It may be seen that after the decontrol of phosphatic and potassic fertilisers, the distortions in NPK ratio has taken place. There has not been any improvement in last 2 years in NPK ratio. This would affect the agricultural productivity in the long run if suitable measures are not taken to reverse the trend.

Table 1.16: N, P, K Ratio during 1952-53 to 1993-94

Year	N	P	K
1952-53	17.5	1.4	1
1961-62	8.9	2.2	1
1971-72	6.0	2.0	1
1981-82	6.0	2.0	1
1986-87	6.7	2.4	1
Kharif 1991	5.4	2.3	1
Rabi 1991-92	6.4	2.6	1
1991-92	5.9	2.4	1
Kharif 1992	6.6	2.5	1
Rabi 1992-93	15.1	4.6	1
1992-93	9.5	3.2	1
Kharif 1993	9.3	2.7	1
Rabi1993-94	10.0	3.2	1
1993-94	9.7	2.9	1
Kharif 1994	9.4	3.0	1
Rabi 1994-95	8.6	2.6	1
1994-95	8.9	2.8	1

Fertiliser Promotion

The essence of "Marketing Concept" is that the customer (farmer) becomes the pivot around which the entire operations of business revolve. Satisfaction of customer becomes the most important goal of business enterprise. Fertiliser industry is conscious of the fact that merely reaching the inputs to the farmers, though important, would not be enough to increase fertiliser use. Convincing him of the efficient use of fertilisers and the economics thereof (particularly with rising prices) and helping him to make farming a profitable venture and not merely a means of subsistence is equally important. With this end in view, the Fertiliser Industry has been playing a vital role in propagating the scientific use of fertilisers and other necessary inputs for higher crop production and productivity. Detailed promotional activities of the industry has been published in April 1996 issue of *Fertiliser News* published by FAI, New Delhi.

Fertiliser Use Scenario in East and North East

East and North-Eastern region has special features and special problems which also need special treatment. Broad soil characteristics, annual rainfall, and irrigated area of the North East region given in Table 1.17 and altitude, temperature and crops grown are given in Table 1.18.

Table 1.17: Broad Soil Characteristics, Annual Rainfall, Nutrient Consumption and Irrigated Area in Eastern Himalayan Region

Zone	Districts (State)	Broad Soil Characteristics	Annual Rainfall (mm)	Nutrient Consumption (1984-85 & 1985-86)			Area Irrigated ('000 ha.)
				N	P_2O_5	K_2O	
NEH Region							
Alpine	Sikkim			6.3	4.9	1.0	
	Himalyan Arunachal Pradesh	Himalayan rock, highly acidic	Above 3000	NA	NA	NA	
	Darjeeling West Bengal			29.9	13.9	15.4	NA
Temperate	Tuenchang (Nagaland)			0.9	0.8	0.1	
Sub-Alpine	Zunenbhuto (Nagaland)	Mountain ranges	Above 3000				
	Mokakchung (Nagaland)						
	Tawang (AP),						
	Bomdilla (AP)						NA
	West Kameng (AP)						
	Shillong (Meghalaya),			8.7	6.5	1.0	
	North & East Manipur,			23.5	6.2	1.0	
	High areas of Sikkim,						
	High areas of Mizoram						
Sub-Tropical	Tirap (AP), Jaintiya and West Garo Hills (Meghalaya), Nonghi Mangao and Gangtok (Sikkim) and Mizoram (except North & South)	Loamy silt Low to Medium in organic low in P and K	1600	NA	NA	NA	NA
Sub-Tropical valley	Imphal (Manipur), Bhagti and Longnak and Jaintia Hills (Meghalaya)	Alluvial soils	Above 2000	NA	NA	NA	NA
Mild Tropical	South Jaintia & North Khasi Hills (Meghalaya), West Manipur Jiribam & Rangpo (Sikkim), Dimapur & Ghaspani (Nagaland), Jampui, Tripura, North Mizoram	Loamy silt, Low in organic matter and P	1400	NA	NA	NA	NA
Mild Tropical Plain	Pasighat, Singhphow and Lohit (AP), West Garo Hills (Meghalaya), Most of Tripura, Dimapur (Nagaland)	Laterite and alluvial soils	2000	NA	NA	NA	NA

Table 1.18: Altitude, Temperature and Crops Grown in Different Zones of NE India

Zones	Altitude Range	Mean Temp. Max.	Mean Temp. Min.	Crop Grown
1. Alpine	More than 3500 m	17°C	0 to 2°C	Natural vegetation pasture.
2. Temperate sub-alpine	1500—3000 m	20°C	0 to 2°C	Shifting cultivation, small millets, potato, rice, maize, barley, minor oilseeds, vegetables.
3. Sub-tropical hill	1000—1500 m	30°C	12°C	Shifting cultivation, rice, maize, wheat, mustard, castor, soybean, pulses, peas, ginger, turmeric.
4. Sub-tropical (Valley area)	400—1000 m	27°C	10°C	Irrigated rice and other crops as above.
5. Mild tropical hill	200—800 m	30°C	12°C	Upland rice, maize, pulses, cotton, wheat.
6. Mild tropical plan	0—200 m	33°C	17°C	Irrigated and rainfed rice, oilseeds, sugarcane, jute and other fibre crops, sweet palio, potato.

The soils of the region are mainly alluvial, lateritic and non-lateritic red soils, and acidic in nature. These are medium to high in N, low to medium in P and medium to high in K status. The soil fertility status varies with soil texture, rainfall intensity, crops grown, flood, slope, and farming methods used. Losses of N by run-off and leaching, and P & K fixation are the common nutritional problems in the region. Though forest and peat soils are high in fertility, they are generally not used for cultivation. Soil erosion in hill slopes and siltation in plains are common features resulting in reduction of top fertile soil layer. Shifting cultivation is still practiced in the region.

Nutrient Balance Sheet

Depleting land fertility due to soil erosion, high intensity rainfall and crop removal, has become a threat to sustainable agriculture in the region. Nutrient removal (by crops and statewise) are mentioned in Table 1.19 and Table 1.20 respectively. Amount of fertiliser nutrient added and nutrient balanced sheet are mentioned (Table 1.21 and Table 1.22). Nutrient addition is much below the recommended dose (Recommended dose of fertiliser in Nagaland is given in Table 1.23).

Table 1.19: Nutrient Removal by Crops in Eastern Himalayan Region

('000 t)

Crop	N	P_2O_5	K_2O	Total
Rice	66.08	19.81	81.96	167.85
Wheat	3.19	0.33	3.35	6.87
Maize	1.19	0.37	2.28	3.84
Millets	0.21	0.08	0.73	1.02
Oilseeds	5.80	2.88	6.02	14.70
Sugar cane	2.33	1.17	3.25	6.75
Cotton	1.16	0.34	2.00	3.50
Jute	9.20	0.07	1.00	10.27
Tea	15.40	1.70	6.80	23.90
Total	104.56	26.75	107.39	238.70

Table 1.20: Statewise Nutrient Removal by Crops

('000 t)

Crop	N	P_2O_5	K_2O	Total
Arunachal Pradesh	3.64	1.16	4.98	9.78
Assam	69.37	19.12	75.51	164.00
Manipur	5.05	1.53	6.38	12.96
Meghalaya	3.86	1.03	4.58	9.47
Mizoram	1.26	0.38	1.70	3.34
Nagaland	2.08	0.71	2.57	5.36
Sikkim	1.32	0.41	1.98	3.71
Tripura	7.93	2.38	9.75	20.06
Total	104.56	26.75	107.39	238.70

Table 1.21: Nutrient Addition in Eastern Himalayan States

('000 t)

States	N		P_2O_5		K_2O		Total	
	1991-92	1994-95	1991-92	1994-95	1991-92	1994-95	1991-92	1994-95
Arunachal Pradesh	0.28	0.23	0.14	0.15	0.05	0.06	0.47	0.44
Assam	19.30	24.49	7.84	4.39	8.39	13.21	35.53	42.09
Manipur	6.15	7.51	2.43	0.88	0.25	0.14	8.83	8.53
Meghalaya	1.53	1.90	1.47	1.12	0.34	0.17	3.33	3.19
Mizoram	0.36	0.18	0.40	0.18	0.04	0.21	0.80	0.57
Nagaland	0.28	0.17	0.35	0.08	0.07	0.00	0.71	0.26
Sikkim	0.95	0.64	0.56	0.29	0.07	0.09	1.58	1.03
Tripura	6.61	4.82	2.58	1.63	1.31	0.98	10.49	7.44
Total	35.46	39.94	15.77	8.72	10.52	14.86	61.74	63.55

Table 1.22: Nutrient Deficit in Eastern Himalayan States

('000 t)

States	N		P_2O_5		K_2O		Total	
	1991-92	1994-95	1991-92	1994-95	1991-92	1994-95	1991-92	1994-95
Arunachal Pradesh	3.36	3.41	1.02	1.01	4.93	4.92	9.31	9.34
Assam	50.07	44.88	11.28	14.73	67.12	62.30	128.47	121.91
Manipur	—	—	—	0.65	6.13	6.24	4.13	6.32
Meghalaya	2.33	1.96	—	—	4.24	4.41	6.14	6.28
Mizoram	0.90	1.08	—	0.20	1.66	1.49	2.54	2.77
Nagaland	1.80	1.91	0.36	0.63	2.50	2.57	4.65	5.10
Sikkim	0.37	0.68	—	0.12	1.91	1.89	2.13	1.29
Tripura	1.32	3.11	—	0.75	8.45	8.78	9.58	12.63
Total	60.15	57.03	12.66	18.09	96.94	92.60	166.95	165.64

Table 1.23: Recommended Fertiliser Dose in Nagaland

State	Kg/ha. as Fertiliser		
	N	P_2O_5	K_2O
Rice	40—50	30—40	20—30
Wheat	45—60	30—40	20—25
Maize	40—60	30—45	20—25
Pigeonpea	20	50	—
Chickpea	20	50	—
Greengram	20	50	—
Blackgram	20	40.50	—
Lentil	20	40—50	—
Sugarcane	150—180	80—90	70—80
Jute			
Capsularis	40	20	20
Olitarius	20	10	10

Constraints

There are various constraints to fertiliser use. These are natural, technological, input related and socio-economical. These constraints need to be solved to increase fertiliser use.

Conclusion

(i) Water control, though not possible as such, may be achieved to some extent with water harvesting and recycling techniques and drainage measures where possible.

(ii) Watershed management approaches and developing rainfed agriculture techniques for higher response to applied nutrients need encouragement.

(iii) Development of need based, problem oriented and situation specific varieties and agro-techniques along with easy and accessible input delivery system to enable timely practices, will definitely enhance nutrient addition to bridge the gap.

(iv) Farmers socio-economic conditions must be raised through adult education programmes, providing sufficient credit and other incentives with easy process and touching all the farmers by transfer of technology programmes.

(v) The region is deficient in foodgrain and has to produce 8.6 mt. foodgrain by 2000 and 22 mt. by 2050 AD. The task ahead is, no doubt stupendous and will not be possible unless productivity is increased to the required level through integrated and balanced use of plant nutrient.

Acknowledgement

Help and services rendered by Dr. S. Das, Agronomist, FAI in preparation of the paper is gratefully acknowledged.

REFERENCES

Bhattacharyya, H.C. and Pathak, A.K., "Fertiliser Use in Eastern Himalayan Region", *Fertiliser News*, 35(6): 15-19 (1990).

Bhattacharyya, H.C. and Pathak, A.K., "Nutrient Balance and Sustainable Agriculture in Eastern Himalayan Region", *Fertiliser News*, 36(6): 19-22 (1991).

Nand, S., *Fertiliser Supply Scenario*, Lecture delivered in Training Programme organised by IFFCO, Phulpur, April 2-3, 1996.

Saxena, S.K., *Fertiliser Marketing Scenario—Retrospect and Prospect*, 5th International Fertiliser Seminar, Amman (Jordan), April 14-19, 1996.

2

INTEGRATED PLANT NUTRIENT SUPPLY SYSTEM (IPNS) AND SUSTAINABLE AGRICULTURE

— *S.K. Saha*

Fertiliser is a vital input in the development of Indian agriculture. "Fertiliser is the food for plants and foodgrain is the food for man". According to FAO and World Bank, the fertiliser use accounts for more than 50 per cent of the total increase in foodgrain production, has contributed significantly in improving the country's food security since mid-1960s. Today India's foodgrain production has reached to a level of 192 million tonnes through use of mainly chemical fertilisers against 50 million tonnes in 1950-51 through mainly organic farming. Similarly, the fertiliser consumption has gone up from only 66,000 tonnes in 1951-52 to 13.52 million tonnes of nutrients in 1994-95 on the one hand and use of fertilisers on the other. However, there is some increase in the area under cultivation from 119.4 million hectares in 1950 to 133.2 million hectares in 1960 to about 143 million hectare at present, larger area being brought under irrigation (from 29.5 million ha. in 1962 to 64 million ha. in 1994), more area under High Yielding Varieties Crops (HYV) from 1.9 million hectare in 1966 to 74.5 million hectare in 1994, support from Agricultural Scientists, Government Departments, Extension Agencies (both Governmental and Non-Governmental). Fertiliser Industries, assistance from National and International Agencies and finally, the hard work put in by the farmers themselves have contributed to this achievement. Dr. Norman Borlaug, the Nobel Laureate, has very rightly said, "If the high yielding varieties of wheat and rice were the catalysts that ignited The Green Revolution, the Chemical Fertilisers were the fuel that powered its forward thrust". However, this is not the end and there will have to be another green revolution as the increasing population has to be supported by farming at almost stabilised net cultivated area. Therefore, higher crop productivity per unit land per unit time through proper farmer's education is of vital interest to million of farmers of the country. Sustainability of Indian agriculture is a key issue of today and the fertiliser use and nutrient balance is a key component of sustainability.

The definitions of sustainable agriculture range from subsistence farming schemes to dynamic systems capable of meeting the needs of growing populations.

Nutritional Security

The country has not achieved food security in real terms so far. Due to over population, unemployment and under-employment, a large section of the society is unable to provide sufficient food to their families. Besides increasing food production, eliminating widespread poverty and improving purchasing power is essential to enable all the people to purchase adequate amount of food. A 33 per cent increase to per capita food consumption would be needed to bring the diet of the present population up to international nutritional standards of calories intake. Nutritional security defined as "physical and economic assets to balanced diet" is still a dream for over two-fifths of the Indian population.

Projected Demand by 2000 AD

India's progress in food production has been overshadowed by rapid population growth. The country's foodgrain demand to feed a population of about 100 crores by 2000 AD is estimated to be around 240 million tonnes. As there seems to be very little scope of expansion in area, the entire increase of about 48 mt in production has to come from increase in productivity. Fertilisers alone will account for over two-thirds of the increase in foodgrains productivity. In the total increase of 48 million tonnes 32 million tonnes has to come from increased use of fertilisers. India's requirement for fertilisers to achieve the targeted foodgrains production of 240 million tonnes is estimated to be around 20 million tonnes. This is over 65 per cent of current consumption and it is doubtful to achieve the same without the government's strong political will and commitment to maintain food security (Table 2.1).

Table 2.1: Some Important Projections by 2000 AD

Particulars	Quantity
Foodgrain Production (mt)	240.0
Nutrient requirement (mt)	28.8
Fertiliser consumption (mt)	17.6
Contribution necessary from other sources (soil : organic and biological) (mt)	11.2

Fertility Status of Soils

The fertility status of soils indicates their nutrient supplying capability. Only a fraction of the total nutrients present in soil exist in readily or potentially usable form on a short-medium terms basis and therefore a knowledge of available nutrient status of soils is very valuable in planning nutrient needs in agriculture. At present, deficiencies of five nutrients are of large scale practical importance in India and therefore much of the focus is on N, P, K, S and Zn. An overall picture of fertility status of soils is provided in Table 2.2.

Table 2.2: Nutrient Status of Indian Soils and the Deficiencies Which Need Attention

Nutrient	Soil Fertility Status
Nitrogen	Low in 228 districts, medium in 118, high in 18 districts.
Phosphorus	Low in 170 districts, medium in 184, high in 17 districts.
Potassium	Low in 47 districts, medium in 192, high in 122 districts.
Sulphur	Deficiencies scattered in 100-120 districts.
Magnesium Zinc	Kerala, other southern states, very acid soils 50% of 150,000 soils analysed found deficient.
Iron	On upland calcareous soils for rice, groundnut, sugarcane.
Boron	Parts of Bihar, Karnataka, West Bengal.

The basic concept underlying IPNS is the maintenance or adjustment of soil fertility and of plant nutrient supply to an optimum level for sustaining the desired crop productivity through optimisation of the benefits from all possible sources of plant nutrients such as chemical fertilisers, organic manures (FYM, Green Manures, Crop Residues), biofertilisers etc. in an integrated manner.

India is the third largest consumer as well as producer and second largest importer of fertilisers in the world (Table 2.3). However, the average per hectare consumption of fertiliser nutrients in India has reached to a level of 74 kg. in 1994-95 as compared to 0.55 kg. in 1951-52, though still it is low, as compared to other countries. The fertiliser consumption and yield of principal crops of some selected countries are given in Table 2.4. China which is the highest user of organic manure in the world also uses relatively higher quantity of chemical fertilisers.

Table 2.3: Production, Import and Consumption of Fertilisers in India during 1994-95
(In million tonnes)

Nutrients	Production	Import	Consumption
N	7.84	1.47	9.51
P_2O_5	2.56	0.38	2.94
K_2O	—	1.28	1.06
Total	10.50	3.13	13.51

Source: Fertiliser Statistics (1994-95), FAI, New Delhi.

Table 2.4: Fertiliser Consumption and Yield of Principal Crops—Some Selected Countries (1993-94)

Name of the Countries	Fertiliser Consumption ($N + P_2O_5 + K_2O$) kg/ha. of arable land	Yield (kg/ha.)			
		Paddy	Wheat	Maize	Patato
India	72.9	2,817	2,420	1,750	15,000
Pakistan	101.0	2,501	1,876	1,450	13,195
Bangladesh	97.8	2,796	1,839	904	10,957
China	261.4	5,869	3,318	5,033	12,505
Japan	407.1	6,770	3,718	2,485	30,357
Phillppines	60.7	3,030	—	1,722	13,060
Korea DPR	315.0	3,507	1,111	3,567	12,052
Korea REP	473.8	6,083	2,857	4,167	20,000
Netherlands	559.9	—	8,067	7,164	45,049
U.K.	338.0	—	7,178	—	41,437
U.S.A.	108.4	6,718	2,526	8,697	37,394
World	83.4	3,651	2,445	4,330	14,591

Source: FAO Production Year Book, Vol. 48, FAO Rome.

As per the estimated figures about 280 million tonnes of composts were produced during 1991-92 which might have added about 2 tonnes of organic manure per hectare. About 6.7 million hectares of area was covered under green manuring.

The present production of Biofertilisers in India is about 2,300 tonnes with estimated achievements of about 39,000 tonnes by 2000 A.D.

It has been mentioned earlier that India is the second largest importer of fertilisers in the world and deficient in fertiliser production (Table 2.3). Plant nutrient removal by crops is much higher than the addition through fertilisers, hence there is a need to promote use of Integrated Plant Nutrient Supply System (IPNS). In this system, judicious use of chemical fertilisers, organic manures and biofertilisers may play a very effective role. This may be supplementary and complementary to each other.

Fertilisers

The fertiliser use grew at slow and steady pace in pre-HYV era. However, in post-HYV era, the growth in fertiliser consumption has been quite rapid (Table 2.5).

Table 2.5: Role of Fertilisers in Increasing Foodgrains Production in India

Year	Fertiliser Consumption (kg/ha)			
	N	P_2O_5	K_2O	Total
1951-52	0.44	0.05	0.06	0.55
1960-61	1.39	0.35	0.19	1.93
1970-71	8.92	3.26	1.43	13.61
1980-81	21.31	7.03	3.61	31.95
1990-91	43.02	17.33	7.14	67.49
1994-95	52.05	16.11	5.83	73.99

Organic Manures

Organic farming system in India is not new and is being followed from ancient times. It improves physical properties of the soil but its nutrient supplying capacity, particularly for HYVs is rather low. Further, its limited availability and transportation is a major constraint for its larger uses. However, it helps in keeping agricultural production at higher level and makes it sustainable.

Biofertilisers

Biofertilisers are a microbial inoculants and are biologically active products consisting of selected strains of viable micro-organisms such as bacteria, algae, fungi, alone or its combination with the ability to fix atmospheric nitrogen or to solubilise plant nutrients like phosphorus and thus rendering them available to plants.

A number of biofertilisers are now available in India. Depending upon the nutrients provided, these can be broadly classified as follow:

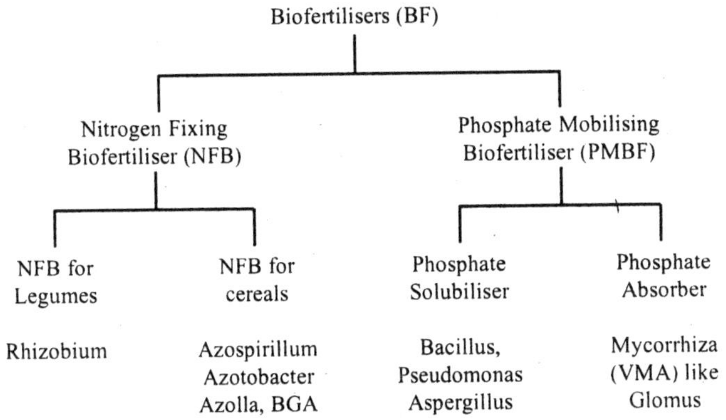

The production of Biofertilisers during 1992-93 was 2,211.8 tonnes (Table 2.6). However, efforts are on to popularise the use of biofertilisers in India. The estimated production target is 39,000 tonnes for 2000 A.D.

Biofertilisers are living organisms and for its proper functioning, optimum environment for storage, transportation, handling and application is a must.

Table 2.6: Production of Biofertiliser during 1992-93

S.No.	Name of the State	Total (in tonnes)
1.	Andhra Pradesh	18.0
2.	Assam	5.0
3.	Gujarat	417.0
4.	Haryana	15.0
5.	Karnataka	27.0
6.	Kerala	4.0
7.	Madhya Pradesh	440.0
8.	Maharashtra	152.0
9.	Manipur	3.0
10.	Meghalaya	0.7
11.	Orissa	35.0
12.	Rajasthan	97.0
13.	Tamil Nadu	863.0
14.	Tripura	—
15.	Uttar Pradesh	125.0
16.	Delhi	4.1
17.	Pondicherry	2.0
	Total	2,211.8

Need for IPNS

It has been mentioned earlier (Table 2.1) that the estimated nutrient removal for the required foodgrain production by 2000 A.D. would be 28.8 million tonnes against the present consumption of 13.52 million tonnes. The nutrient supply through fertiliser is expected to be 17.6 million tonnes by 2000 A.D. Therefore, a deficit of 11.2 million tonnes would have to be met from sources other than fertilisers. These sources include contribution from soil, organic manure, biofertilisers, etc.

Conclusion

Although the crop response to organic and biofertilisers are not as spectacular as with chemical fertilisers, but the complementary and supplementary use of organic and biofertilisers, besides improving soil properties also improves the efficiency of applied fertilisers. Hence in India IPNS is the only answer for achieving sustainability in agriculture.

3

INTEGRATED NUTRIENT MANAGEMENT IN FRUIT CROPS

— *P.L. Kar*

Preamble

India occupies a place of pride in the world scenario of fruit production ranking the first position. But the level of productivity at present is only 12.36 tonnes/ha which is quite low and has to be brought to international level of 40 tonnes/ha. This invariably will entail use of appropriate quantities of N : P_2O_5 : K_2O with other inputs as per recommended ratio of 0.75 : 0.50 : 1.00. The requirement of 0.67 million tonnes N, 0.46 million tonnes P_2O_5 and 0.91 million tonnes of K_2O as per the above ratio has to be raised to 1.07, 0.58 and 1.14 million tonnes, respectively by the turn of 2000 A.D. to supply the recommended dose of fertiliser nutrients to an area of 3.64 million ha under fruit cultivation (Yadav, 1999).

Fertility and Increase Productivity of Soil

In the known Indian history from 500 B.C., Indian soils supported many kingdoms which flourished and perished resulting in impoverished soils over centuries. Before independence, farmers survived with extensive cultivation and low yields. After independence, substantial investments were made in creating various infrastructure facilities and developed various need based inputs to set the stage for higher yields. However, under intensive agriculture to support high yields, high inputs of plant nutrients are invariably needed. In the post-independence era, conventional organic manures, oil cakes, green manures alone could not meet the nutritional needs of high yielding crop varieties. The fertiliser consumption increased from a mere 0.07 million tonnes in 1950-51 to huge amount of about 16.2 million tonnes in 1997-98 (Rao and Srivastava, 1999). Even, with the use of such a large amount of fertilisers in the country, soil fertility in respect of N and P has not increased and remained low or medium in status. But soils in pockets of areas in some states might have got enriched with P. The deficiencies of K, S, Zn, Fe, B, etc. have been fast increasing in time and space (Rao and Srivastava, 1998). Indian farmers, not alarmed at the declining soil fertility, continue to exploit soil resources with only marginal replenishments.

Fertility Status of Indian Soil

Fruit crops are heavy feeder of plant nutrients, removing 200-1,500 kg. of N, P and K per ha (Yadav, 1999). Papaya, grape and banana are heavy feeders of K. Although recommended dose of K_2O for banana is only 728 kg/ha, a good crop is known to remove 1,000 kg or more K_2O from 1 ha. The annual gap between nutrient additions and removal is of the order of 9-10 million tonnes (Biswas *et al.*, 1998). Since the nutrient additions have never kept pace with nutrient removal by crops and cropping system, the fertility status of Indian soils is fast declining. As crops remove huge quantities of K from soil and the amounts of fertiliser K applied are small, the maintenance of fertility of Indian soils with respect to K and safeguarding higher productivity of the crops in future may become a big task (Subba Rao *et al.*, 1993).

In India, 5 plant nutrient elements, namely N, P, K, S and Zn are of widespread practical importance. The nutrient status of Indian soil with respect to nitrogen, phosphorus, potassium and secondary and micro-nutrients is shown in Table 3.1.

Table 3.1: Nutrient Status of Soils in India (400 Districts)

Nutrient	Category	No. of Blocks	
Nitrogen	Low—228	Medium—118	High—18
Phosphorus	Low—170	Medium—184	High—17
Potassium	Low—47	Medium—194	High—122
Sulphur	Deficiencies scattered in 130 districts		
Magnesium	Kerala, other Southern states, very acidic soils		
Zinc	50% of 200,000 soil analysed found deficient		
Iron	Important on upland calcareous soils		
Boron	Parts of Bihar, West Bengal and Karnataka		

Further imbalance application of N (due to its low price) neither increases yield nor the profit in the long run. But it may result in accelerating deficiency of other nutrients in the soil. Experimental evidences suggest that N alone in different crop sequence at various locations in the country increased depletion of available P from the soil, thus causing fast appearance of P deficiency. The same is true for other plant nutrients. This calls for avoidance of the practice.

Soil Fertility and Fertiliser Management

Good soil fertility means good crop yield. Preventing the loss of plant nutrients from an ecosystem is important for soil fertility management. Nitrogen, phosphorus and potassium (N, P, K) are the three major elements which determine soil fertility and should be ideally present in 4 : 2 : 1; abberations affect fertility and therefore yield. Urea, containing 46 per cent of N, is applied to crop in largest amount but less than half of this N, in the form of nitrate, is available to crops. The rest is lost through 'leaching' or by 'volatilisation' or by surface run-off after a heavy shower. Leaching of soluble nitrates into the sub-soil and eventually into ground water can go to the extent of 50 to 70 per cent. Leaching not only depletes precious nitrates but also takes away clay, soil and organic matter leading to low chemical soil fertility and low plant available water resources. Ammonia volatilisation also can contribute to nearly 60 per cent nitrate loss. Loss through volatilisation occurs when denitrifying bacterial reduce the nitrate to elemental nitrogen and nitrous oxide which escape to the stratosphere and cause ozone depletion accompanied by environmental warning.

Similarly, availability of phosphorus to crops from applied phosphatic fertiliser under soils with acidic reaction is extremely low and bulk of the phosphate get lost due to complex chelate formation. It is a common issue that different plant nutrients applied to crops for growth and production are not available in full and a reckonable percentage of the elements is lost. This in terms of financial scale will be a loss of great magnitude which our farmers and the country can hardly afford.

Nutrition and Nutrient Management in Fruit Crops

The need of mineral nutrition and nutrient management in fruit trees differ from those of annual crops in number of ways mentioned as below:

- Fruit trees have a long pre-bearing period.
- Requirement of nutrients vary with age of the plant.

— Generally, they have a deep root system and remain at the same place for years together which calls for regular monitoring of soil.
— Fruit crops have distinct and lengthy phases of vegetative and reproductive development.
— There is a need to supply nutrient continuously for a current production as well as for the vegetative reserve in perennial crops, which persist for several years.

The nutrient requirements of fruit crops in respect of N, P and K based on the recommended dose are presented in Table 3.2.

Table 3.2: Area, Recommended Dose and Nutrient Requirement of Fruits

Fruit	Area (ha)	Recommended Doses			National Fertiliser Requirement		
		N (kg/ha)	P_2O_5 (kg/ha)	K_2O (kg/ha)	N (tonnes)	P_2O_5 (tonnes)	K_2O (tonnes)
Mango	11,36,668	50	30	63	56,833	34,100	71,610
Banana	3,96,197	504	366	728	1,99,683	1,45,008	2,88,431
Citrus	3,69,588	190	104	160	70,216	38,434	59,129
Apple	1,91,203	108	109	210	20,650	20,847	40,164
Guava	1,11,851	115	81	145	12,863	9,060	16,218
Pineapple	59,436	424	115	372	25,201	6,835	22,110
Litchi	53,561	245	395	615	13,122	21,157	32,940
Papaya	47,429	434	434	868	20,584	20,584	41,129
Grape	34,010	648	419	867	22,038	14,250	29,487
Sapota	30,777	100	60	102	3,078	1,847	3,170
Others	7,74,906	300	200	400	2,43,472	1,54,981	3,09,962
Total	3,2,05,596	—	—	—	8,62,472	4,67,103	9,14,389

Source: I.S. Yadav (1999) Ind. Hort.
Total of N + P_2O_5 + K_2O fertiliser required = 22,44,088 tonnes.

Based on the area (3.21 million ha), production (31.48 million tonnes) and recommended doses of fertilisers for various fruit crops, the projected current requirement of N, P_2O_5 and K_2O together at 700 kg of N + P_2O_5 + K_2O per ha, will be 2.24 million tonnes annually, constituting nearly 17.2 per cent of the total fertiliser used in the country. With the targeted figure of enhancing the productivity, further increase in the use of fertilisers to 800 kg/ha has been envisaged during 2000 A.D. which will involve a total use of 2.80 million tonnes of fertiliser.

Integrated Nutrient Supply and Management in Fruit Crops

For realising high yield of fruit crops, soil health has to play a paramount role. The low yield of fruit crops in our country is associated with the low and deteriorating soil fertility. The disproportionate use of fertiliser has widen soil imbalance in terms of NPK ratio. A national assessment of nutrient efficiency reveals that (1) Nitrogen deficiency is universal and would continue to be so. (2) Nearly 49, 20, 47 per cent of Indian soil are deficient in phosphorus, potassium and zinc, respectively. (3) Potassium deficiency becomes most limiting factor for crop production and iron management. Manganese, Boron and Sulphur will affect the productivity in majority of Indian soil. Besides, it is also estimated that every year nearly 8 million tonnes of nutrients are depleted.

The concept of Integrated Nutrient Management Programme (INMP) refers to combined use of mineral fertiliser, organic manure, green manuring, biofertilisers (Rhizobium, N fixers, P solubilisers) and crop residues with the objective of obtaining high yields and ensuring environmental safety. The INSP aims at sustainable productivity with minimum deleterious effect of chemical fertilisers on soil health and environment.

Components of Integrated Nutrient Supply Programme (INSP)

Under INSP the nutrients are desired to be supplied from various sources to make them affordable to the farmers and at the same time sustainable. These may be critically viewed as under:

Organic Manure

Usefulness of FYM increasing fruit crop yield when combined with mineral fertiliser is well documented. However, the point of consideration is about availability of FYM/compost to meet the large nutrient requirements of all agricultural and horticultural crops. Growers must use FYM as a supplemental source rather than as substitution of nutrients through fertilisers. According to an estimate, the availability of the resource is:

Table 3.3: Availability of Organic Manures

Cattle dung	2 billion tonnes
Urban compost	6.64 mt
Rural compost	279.66 mt
Area under green manure	6.71 m.ha. (1991-92)

Source: Balanced Fertiliser use for Sustainable Agriculture in India. Potash and Phosphate Institute of Canada, India Programme, Gurgaon-122 016, Haryana.

Modern technology for increased production does not mean that bulky organic manure, etc. should be ignored. Organics are useful sources for supply of nutrients and have many other advantages when applied in soil. Therefore, combined use of organic manures and inorganic fertilisers need to be encouraged. However, in the process, fertiliser will continue to be the dominant contributor for meeting plant nutrient requirements of crops for increasing production.

Importance of Micro-nutrients

Shift in fertiliser consumption pattern from low to high and more chemically pure fertilisers has caused deficiency of secondary and micro-nutrient in soils. Increases in yield of crops with sulphur application have also been recorded. Among various micro-nutrients essential for plants, deficiency of zinc has become a major problem in many parts of the country. Non-application of micro-nutrients in areas where deficiencies of these nutrients exist affects even the efficiency of NPK fertilisers resulting in poor crop yields.

Nutrient balance must be considered beyond N, P and K ignoring deficiencies of secondary and/or micro-nutrients in the soil results in significant losses in yield and in efficiency of applied NPK. Therefore, it is necessary to identify all deficient plant nutrients and develop a balanced fertilisation programme to offset their effect as yield limiting factors.

Biofertilisers

Biofertilisers are micro-organisms which are capable of mobilising nutritive elements from non-usable form through biological process. They are cost-effective and inexpensive source of plant nutrients, do not require non-renewable source of energy during their production, improve crop growth and quality of the products by producing plant hormones, help in sustainable crop production through maintenance of soil productivity. They are useful as bio-control agents, since they control many plant pathogen and harmful micro-organisms.

Biofertilisers are not alternatives for inorganic fertilisers. But they are useful in increasing yield, quality and production of crops when they are used in combination with organic manure and inorganic fertiliser in a balanced proportion. The biofertilisers that can be used in horticulture are nitrogen fixers, phosphate solubilisers and mycorrhizal fungi (Mohandas, 1999).

The nitrogen fixing organisms for horticultural crops are *Rhizobium* sp., *Azospirillum* sp. and *Azotobacter* sp. Phosphate-solubilising micro-organisms are soil bacteria particularly *Pseudomonas* and *Becillus* and fungal *Penicillum* and *Aspergillus* sp. They possess ability to bring insoluble phosphates in soil into soluble forms by secreting organic acids such as acetic, formic, propionic, laetic, glycolic, fumeric and succinic acids. These acids lower pH and bring about dissolution of bound form of phosphate. *Mycorrhizal* fungi are most common fungal association among angiosperm. The vesicular-arbuscular mycorrhizae (VAM) are formed which are beneficial to plant when they colonise. They make more nutrient available to plant, improve soil texture, water holding capacity, improve disease resistance and help in better plant growth. Besides, they are helpful in biological control of root pathogens.

Papaya, litchi, mango, citrus, banana, grape and pomegranate are all benefited by the VAM inoculation.

Table 3.4: Nutrients Fixed/made Available by Different Micro-organisms

Micro-organism	Associated with	Dose (kg./ha./year)
Rhizobium fixing	Leguminous vegetables	30—180
Azospirillum and *Azotobacter* N-fixing	Non-leguminous vegetables	30—80
Phosphate-solubilising micro-organisms	Transplantable vegetables and fruits	Solubilises 40—100 of fixed P
Mycorrhiza	All vegetable and fruit crops	

Source: Sukhada Mohandas (1999). *Ind. Horticulture*, 1999.

Table 3.5: Biofertilisers for Horticultural Crops

Fruit	Micro-organisms	Method of Application
Mango, citrus, Papaya, banana, grape, litchi and pomegranate	VAM fungi, Glomus mosseae, *G. fasciculatum*, *Azospirillum* and phosphate-solubilising bacteria.	Nursery application and to be applied in pits while transplanting.

Source: Sukhada Mohandas (1999) *Ind. Horticulture*.

Fertiliser Use Efficiency in INSP

The cost of input is very high. Further losses of expensive fertiliser due to leaching, biological processes, chemical fixation, erosion, volatilisation, etc. in occasions are high. Minimisation of losses and increasing the use efficiency of fertiliser in the approach of integrated nutrient management will be extremely crucial to sustain investment and productivity. Efficient management of fertiliser use can be achieved by the application of need-based secondary and micro-nutrients. Urea is the dominant 'N' source for plant nutrition and, as already stated, undergoes losses due to the processes like leaching, volatilisation, surface run-off, hydrolysis, ammonification, etc. thereby reducing the use efficiency of the fertiliser. The key issue of integrated nutrient management practices entails that the use efficiency of the nutrients from various sources should be of the highest order to sustain soil fertility and achieve maximum productivity.

One way to minimise nitrate loss is to apply the urea more than one in smaller quantities or alternatively, to use a 'slow-release urea' which makes the urea available in the soil for a longer time. General ways in which release rates can be controlled are: (1) the application of low solubility coatings to soluble fertiliser, (2) the manufacture of compounds with low solubility, (3) the manufacture of low solubility compounds which in addition require microbial activity for release of the nutrient and (4) treated, natural organic materials which require microbial action for release of nutrients. Brief descriptions of controlled-release fertilisers and their use in horticulture are shown in Table 3.6.

Ammonia volatilisation, urea hydrolysis and leaching were all reduced when urea was blended or coated with neem cake. Similarly, use of nitrification inhibitors can greatly reduce the loss of urea through ammonia volatilisation. On the whole factors contributing to the losses of nutrients should be prevented to derive maximum benefit from their use.

Conclusion

Adequate and balanced nutrient use is the key to increase crop productivity which in turn increases fruit/seed yield per unit of applied nutrient. It will, therefore, be highly pertinent to determine the nutrient imbalances in the soil and apply required amount of nutrients to correct imbalances and optimise crop nutrition. Correction of soil condition, i.e., acidity, sodicity, etc. before application of soil test based fertiliser dose is must to realise the full benefit from the applied fertiliser inputs. Integrated nutrient supply system can help to provide balanced nutrition, sustain crop productivity and arrest fall in factor productivity. To mitigate the deficiencies of S, Zn, Mn, Fe and B, wherever manifested, need-based application of fertiliser materials containing these nutrients need

Table 3.6: Characteristics of Some Controlled-release Fertilisers

Concept Governing Availability	Material	Nutrients Supplied	Typical Analysis	Influence of Environment of Availability			Span of Effectiveness
				Temperature	Moisture	pH	
Costing of a soluble material	SCU	N, S	36% N 17% S	Increases with temperature	Increases with soil moisture	None	Variable, approximately 1% day
	Osmocote	N, P, K	14-6.3-11.6 18-2.7-10	Increases with temperature	Not affected between wilting and field capacity	None	3 to 4 months 8 to 9 months
Low solubility material	IBDU	N	31% N	Increases with temperature	Increases with soil moisture	Greater at low pH, maximum at pH 4	58% in 21 weeks for 1.0 to 1.2 mm particles
	Mag Amp	N, P, Mg	8-17.5-0.14	Slight increase with temperature	Increases with soil moisture	Greater at low pH	100 days for incorporated coarse granules
Low solubility, biodegradable material	Ureaform	N	38% N	Increases with temperature	Maximum at 50% saturation	Maximum at pH 6.1	60% in 6 months for 75% insoluble material with 60 AI
	Activated sludge (Milorganite)	N, P, K	6-1.35-0	Increases with temperature	Increases with soil moisture	Maximum at pH 6-7	2-4 months

to be applied for obtaining sustainable higher yields. Moderate rates of application of organic manures and green manuring can also, to great extent, alleviate the constraints of micro and secondary nutrients and maintain higher yields on long term basis. Arresting the various losses of applied nitrogen and harnessing the residual phosphorus left in the soil by the previous crop through efficient management practices will promote better utilisation of applied nutrients and improve response ratios.

The strategy for sustenance of soil fertility and maintenance of higher production have to be resorted through the work on integrated nutrient management involving organic manures, mineral and biofertilisers for enhancing the nutrient use efficiency need to be continued.

REFERENCES

Anonymous (1996), "Balanced Fertiliser Use for Sustainable Agriculture in India", Potash and Phosphate Institute of Canada, India Programme, Gurgaon-122 016, Haryana, pp. 1-11.

Bhargava, B.S. (1999), "Leaf Analysis for Diagnosing Nutrients Need in Fruit Crops", *Ind. Hort.*, 43 (4): 6-8.

Biswas, B.C.; Prasad, N. and Das, S. (1993), *Fert. News*, 43 (4): 17-20 & 23-30.

Maronek, D.M.; Hendrix, J.W. and Kierman, J. (1981), "Mycorrhizal Fungal and Their Importance in Horticultural Crop Production", *Hort. Review*, 3: 172-213.

Mohandas, S. (1999), "Biofertilisers for Horticulture Crops", *Ind. Hort.*, 43(4): 32-35.

Pandey, A.K. and Singh, K.P. (1998), *Vegetable Production Technology: Towards Productivity Enhancement*, National Symposium, Emerging Scenario in Vegetable Research and Development held on 12-14 December 1998 at PDVR, Varanasi, pp. 77-84.

Saxena, R.C. (1996), Agricultural Technologies for 21st Century: Neem for Sustainable Agriculture and Environmental Conservation, Paper presented at Annual Sustainable Development Conference held in Islamabad, August 4-9, 1996.

Subba Rao, A.; Rao, S. and Ganeshmurthy (1993), *Fert. News*, 38 (12): 61-69.

Subba Rao, A. and Srivastava, S. (1998), *Fert. News*, 43 (4): 65-67.

Subba Rao, A. and Srivastava, S. (1999), "Experiences on Current Status of Crop Response to Fertilisers in Different Agro-climatic Zones" as Learnt from All India Coordinated Research Project on Soil Test Crop Response Correlation, *Fert. News*, 44 (4): 83-95.

Yadav, I.S. (1999), "Nutrient Management in Horticultural Crops", *Ind. Hort.*, 43 (4): 4-5.

4

INTEGRATED NUTRIENT MANAGEMENT IN VEGETABLE CROPS

— V.B. Singh

The vegetable production of our country before independence was merely 15 million tonnes and it increased from 23.45 million tonnes in 1961-65 to 28.36 million tonnes in 1967-71 and to 39.99 million tonnes in 1986. According to latest report, vegetables are grown in 6.2 million ha with a production of 71 million tonnes having 2.6 per cent annual growth.

Thus, in past three decades, India has made a quantum jump in vegetable production, securing the second position in the world. However, this amount is much less than our requirement and serve per capita intake of vegetables only 210 g against the requirement of 285 g per capita per day for balanced diet. There is need to achieve the target of 100 million tonnes for the supply of 250 g vegetables per day per capita to our estimated population of 1 billion by 2000 AD. However, our demand by 2020 AD will be around 250 million tonnes. Besides, to avail our internal demand, vegetables are now being considered as one of the most potential commodities for export. The value of fresh, canned and dehydrated vegetable export has been the tune of Rs. 363.44 crores during 1996-97.

Population growth and urbanisation are creating increased demand of food over and there is growing concern over malnutrition, especially in semi-urban areas. To meet the full dietary needs of common man, to eliminate malnutrition, deficiency diseases and to relieve overstress on cereals, there is greater need of enhanced vegetable production. Among the various factors of production of vegetables, nutrient management is more important with regard to sustain the production and productivity.

For enhancing high yields of vegetable crops, soil health is crucial factor. Unfortunately, deteriorating soil fertility is principally responsible for low yield of vegetables in our country. The disappropriate use of fertiliser has widened soil imbalance in terms of NPK ratio. A nation-wide assessment of nutrient efficiency reveals that (1) Nitrogen deficiency is universal and will continue to be so. (2) Nearly 49, 20 and 47 per cent of Indian soil are deficient in phosphorus, potassium and Zinc respectively. (3) Potassium deficiency becomes most limiting factor for crop production and iron management. Manganese, Boron and Sulphur will affect the productivity in majority of Indian soils. Besides, it was also estimated that every year nearly 8 million tonnes of nutrients are depleted.

Given the situation and the pressure to increase productivity through high nutrient availability and management of costly inorganic fertilisers which is based on non-renewable and exhaustible petroleum based resource. It has now been realised that the use of chemical fertiliser must be integrated through more economic, renewable and environmental-friendly organic fertilisers, biofertilisers, crop residues and green manures.

In simple terms, IPNS is a balance use of chemical fertilisers, organic manure, such as the farm yard manure (FYM), crop residues, animal and human waste, biofertilisers. Recommendations have been made for adopting and strengthening of IPNS during the ninth plan. The IPNS aims at sustainable productivity with minimum deleterious effect of chemical fertilisers on soil health and environment.

Major Nutrient Management

To achieve the self-sufficiency in the vegetable production for growing population of the country, application of chemical fertilisers cannot be ruled out. The potato, onion, tomato and cauliflower contributing about 63 per cent of total vegetable production in our country. They are heavy feeder of plant nutrients requiring N + P_2O_5 + K_2O from 146 to 80 kg/ha and producing 20 to 70 tonnes of vegetables per hectare (recommended dose and nutrient requirement shown in Table 4.1).

On application of recommended dose of primary nutrients to various vegetable crops 12,52,250 tonnes of N + P_2O_5 + K_2O will be required, which is 9.13 per cent of total fertiliser consumption in the country for all agricultural, horticultural land plantation crops. However, the best fertiliser used ratio is 1.3 : 0.80 : 1 for quality vegetable production.

Nitrogen Fertiliser

Nitrogen is a mobile nutrient both in the soil and within the plant.

Table 4.1: Area, Recommended Doses (kg/ha) and Annual Nutrient Requirement (tonnes) of Vegetables

Vegetable	Recommended Doses			Nutrient Requirement			
	N	P_2O_5	K_2O	N	P_2O_5	K_2O	Total
Potato	125	80	100	157,490	100,793	125,992	384,275
Onion	87	50	62	33,118	19,033	23,601	75,752
Tomato	76	47	42	23,458	14,507	12,963	50,928
Cabbage	118	67	74	252,472	14,463	15,974	55,909
Cauliflower	108	55	38	24,072	12,234	8,452	44,709
Okra	100	54	59	28,162	15,208	16,616	59,986
Peas	90	46	87	17,474	8,931	16,819	43,296
Others	100	60	80	223,915	134,349	1,791,323	537,396
Total	100	57	68	533,112	319,518	399,621	1,252,251

Hence, emphasis should be given during the crop duration of each vegetable that the number of split application and time of each application should be manipulated to achieve maximum utilisation and minimum loss of the applied fertiliser. Nitrogen use efficiency of varies considerably among the vegetables depending upon the crop duration and crop characteristics. Out of the six important vegetables: tomato and onion depend more on applied nitrogen whereas the brinjal, okra, french bean absorb more of soil nitrogen. Recovery of applied nitrogen fertiliser ranges from 13.9 per cent in chillies to 44 per cent in brinjal.

Onion has highest physiological efficiency (edible part produced/unit of nitrogen absorbed), whereas brinjal has highest agronomic efficiency (edible part produced/applied) (Table 4.2).

When vegetables are grown intensively, it is necessary to identify efficient cropping sequence. Of the six cropping sequences given in Table 4.2 french bean, tomato-onion and okra-cabbage-brinjal are considered better.

During the crop cultivation—nitrogen fertiliser should be applied in adequate number of split applications and each application should be properly timed.

It is advisable to reduce the proper doses of nitrogen applied in basal dose also to defer its applications by about 10 days after planting causing to improve its use by the vegetable crops and to avoid leaching and volatilisation losses.

The remaining nitrogen fertiliser may be top dressed as in 2 to 3 splits depending upon the crop duration and nature of crop to save 25 per cent of nitrogen fertilisation.

Table 4.2: Uptake of Nitrogen and Nitrogen-Use Efficiency of Vegetable Crops

Crop	N Uptake (kg/ha)		Recovery of Applied N (%)	PE	AE
	Fertiliser	Soil			
French bean (Arka Komal)	22.3	70.5	27.9	150	175
Okra (Pusa Sawani)	46.7	171.6	38.9	220	401
Tomato (Arka Vikas)	42.7	56.8	26.4	513	340
Brinjal (Arka Shirish)	53.4	101.8	44 7	223	844
Onion (Arka Kalyan)	46.1	37.1	25.4	626	289
Chilli (Arka Lohit)	16.7	81.8	13.9	166	137

Phosphatic Fertiliser

Phosphorus is relatively immobile in the soil hence it should be banded to minimise fixation. Binding at proper depth markedly enhance the application of phosphatic fertilisers.

In shallow rooted vegetables like brinjal, chilly, french bean, onion, tomato, placement of superphosphate 5 cm below the seed/plant result in maximum utilisation of applied phosphorus. As a result saving of 50 per cent in brinjal and 20 per cent in onion and tomato is possible. In the deep rooted vegetables like okra placement at 10 cm depth is found superior for effective utilisation of phosphorus (Table 4.3). The water soluble form (superphosphate) is generally fixed in highly acidic soils, and availability of phosphorus in the soil of North-Eastern hill region is

Table 4.3: Comparison of Different Levels of Phosphorus Banded at 5 cm. below the Seed/Plant Row

Level of P_2O_5 (kg/ha)	Recommended Phosphorus (%)	Yield (tonnes/ha)	Fertiliser P	
			Uptake (kg/ha)	Utilisation (%)
(1)	(2)	(3)	(4)	(5)
Tomato				
60	80	23.81b*	5.74	21.94b
75	100	19.50a	5.33	16.27a
Brinjal				
24	60	6.41	2.61	24.89b
40	100	7.10	2.44	13.94a
Onion				
40	80	63.43	4.79	22.95
60	100	65.65	4.86	18.63

(Contd.)

Table 4.3 (*Contd.*)

(1)	(2)	(3)	(4)	(5)
Chilli				
48	60	13.09	5.54	26.54
80	100	17.98	7.17	20.61
Cabbage (Pride of India)				
48	60	9.01	8.97	40.11
80	100	9.34	12.27	35.26
Cabbage (Mahyco Hybrid 412)				
72	60	14.20	14.45	46.15b
120	120	14.35	17.52	33.59a

* The number followed by the same alphabet are not statistically different (P = 0.05) in each crop.

less due to this fact. Hence basic slag, raw and steamed bone meal, rock phosphate are best sources of phophorus for the acid soils of this region.

Potassic Fertiliser

The potassic fertilisers intermediate in mobility in the soil and usually applied along with the basal dose at sowing/planting. Plants take most of their potash requirement in the early stage of their growth. However, split applications may be adopted in long durations on vegetable crops, like chilli, capsicum and indeterminate tomato for best utilisation. It is better to apply them as near as possible to the actively absorbing root zone.

Micro-nutrients Management

The micro-nutrients, namely boron, manganese, iron, molybdenum and copper play an important role in vegetable production. Vegetables like onion, carrot, brassica and sugar beets have high boron requirements. Boron is effective in controlling the malady of total soluble solid ascorbic acid and flesh appearance. Almost all soils producing vegetables are found to deficient in S and Zn. Hence, application of S @10 kg/ha (100 kg superphosphate will supply 11 kg S along with 16 kg P_2O_5); and Zn @10 kg/ha (50 kg Zinc sulphate/ha) will enhance the efficiency of primary nutrients. High rainfall received on light textured soil such as found in southern and coastal Karnataka, Kerala, North-Eastern region of the country, are reported deficient in Mg and need application of either magnesium containing fertilisers such as magnesium sulphate @100 kg/ha or dolomite limestone (Table 4.4).

Table 4.4: Micronutrient Demand of Some of the Vegetables

Boron	Copper	Manganese	Molybdenum	Zinc
Sugar beet	Beet	Sugar beet	Cauliflower	Beans
Turnip	Lettuce	Pea	Lettuce	Cauliflower
Ruta baga	Spinach	Beans	Spinach	
Cauliflower	Carrot	Lettuce		
Brussels	Onion	Spinach		

Organic Farming

In vegetable production, rate of organic manure is much more as compared to other cereal crops. It has been proved experimentally that vegetables produced by the application of organic manure possess good firmness and have long storage life. Now-a-days, vegetables produced by organic system, fetching better price in international as well as in national markets. Organic farming is not for only to produce food of high nutritional quality in sufficient quantity but also to maintain and increase long term fertility of soil to encourage and enhance biological cycles within the farming system involving micro-organisms. It helps towards as far as possible with materials and substances that can be removed or recycled either on farm or elsewhere, thus minimise pollution that may result from agricultural practices. The organic farming provides opportunities for sustainable development and helps in maintaining the genetic diversity of the agricultural systems and its surroundings, including the protection of plants and wildlife and habitats. It is high time, the role of those creatures is fully appreciated so as to make use of them solving the problems of deteriorating soil conditions, meeting nutrient needs and dispersing obnoxious materials.

Organic amendments in form of oil cakes and neem, mahua, GNC and castor suppress the population of nematodes and other harmful pathogens like Fusarium and Rhizoctonia, etc. besides improving soil productivity and enhancing the vegetable production.

Biofertilisers

Recently, application of biofertilisers in vegetable crops has been found very effective. Biofertilisers are micro-organisms which are capable of mobilising nutrient elements from non-usable form to usable form through biological process. They are cost effective and inexpensive source of plant nutrients, do not require non-renewable source of energy during their production, improve crop growth and quality of the products by producing plant hormones, help in sustainable crop production through maintenance of soil productivity. They are useful as bio-control agents, since they control many plant pathogens and harmful micro-organisms.

Table 4.5: Estimated Requirement of Micronutrient and Organic Manures

Micronutrients/Biofertilisers/Organic Manures	Quality	
Zinc sulphate	60,000	tonnes
Borax	30,000	tonnes
Rhizobium	400	tonnes
Azospirillum	155	tonnes
Compost	6,200	lakh tonnes
Digested sludge	6,200	lakh tonnes

Biofertilisers harper atmospheric nitrogen with the help specialised soil micro-organisms are either free living in soil and symbiotic with plants and directly or indirectly contribute towards the nitrogen nutrition of the plants. In onion, inoculation with *Azospirillum brasilens* sp. Nov. and VAM at nursery stage and in the main field recorded an additional yield of 22.93 t/ha and saved 25 per cent recommended dose of NPK fertilisers (Table 4.5).

REFERENCES

Kotur, S.C. and Keshava Murthy, S.V. (1999). "Fertiliser Management in Vegetable Crops", *Indian Horticulture*, 43:4: 23-25.

Mohandas, Sukhada, (1999). *Biofertilisers for Horticultural Crops., Ind. Hort.*, 42(4): 32-35.

Pandey, A.K. and Singh, K.P. (1998). *Vegetable Production Technology: Towards Productivity Enhancement*, Souvenir, Indian Society of Vegetable Science, PDVR, Varanasi, pp. 76-84.

Singh, Kirti (1998). *Challenges in Vegetable Production in 21st Century*, Memorial lecture at National Symposium on Emerging Scenario in Vegetable Research and Development, 12-14 December 1998, PDVR, Varanasi.

Singh, N.P., Singh, A.K. and Singh, V.B. (1998). *Organic Farming in North East India—Prospective for Planning and Development in North East India.*

Singh, V.B., Singh, N.P. and Changkhog, Y. (1995). *Effect of Organic Manures and Methods of Nitrogen Application on the Growth Yield and Quality of Ginger*. In "Proceeding of II Congress of Traditional Science & Technology of India", *Agr. Ho.*, Vol. I, 6-24.

Singh, V.B. (1990). *Fruits of North East Region*, Wiley Eastern Ltd., Daryaganj, New Delhi.

Singh, V.B. and Singh, Kirti (1996). *Spices of India*, New Age International Publication, Daryaganj, New Delhi.

Yadav, I.S. (1999). "Nutrient Management in Horticultural Crops", *Indian Horticulture*, 43(4): 4-5.

5

Integrated Plant Nutrient Supply Systems in Transplanted Rice with Special Reference to North East Region

— *D.N. Medhi, B. Deka Medhi* and *A.C. Sharma*

Fertilisers are the "King Pin" and the costliest input in the present system of crop production. On the other hand, the fertilisers use efficiency on transplanted rice, particularly nitrogen is only 30 to 50 per cent (Prasad and De Datta, 1979). Because losses of fertiliser nutrients take place under submerged condition by different ways. Therefore, the strategy for increasing the efficiency of fertiliser nutrients should include the supplementation of fertiliser nutrients in conjunction with organic resources.

The basic principles of integrated nutrient management system is the maintenance of soil fertility, sustainable agricultural productivity and improving profitability through the judicious and efficient use of mineral fertilisers, organic manures, green manures and biofertilisers etc. The important task of integrated nutrient management is the efficient management of inherent soil fertility.

Potential Organic Resources

The potential organic resources most commonly used to improve soil condition and fertility are excreta of livestock, human beings, crop residues, water hyacinth, sewage and sludge, agro industry wastes, microbial resources, biological resources such as azolla, blue green algae, rhizobia, azotobacter, green manures, etc.

Availability of Nutrients

The benefit of organic manures are generally interpreted in terms of capacity to substitute for inorganic fertiliser, more particularly nitrogen. The factors affecting the nutrients release from the applied organic manures depend upon:

(a) Soil type
(b) Submergence period, i.e. availability of water
(c) Soil temperature
(d) Type of organic manure, its nature and amount
(e) C : N ratio
(f) Lignin content
(g) Method of application.

In an experiment at Assam Agricultural University, Jorhat, DekaMedhi and Medhi (1999) reported that exchangeable NH_4^+–N release was delayed when green manures were added whereas with the addition of urea the peak was reached at 20 days after transplanting (Fig. 5.1) in both the seasons. However, *Sesbania rostrata* released higher NH_4^+–N than did *Sesbania aculeata*. In another experiment, incorporation of organic and inorganic sources of N increased soil and soil solution NH_4^+–N to a peak and then declined to a very low level. Prilled urea gave higher NH_4^+–N than did organic sources at 2 weeks after flooding whereas the reverse trend was obtained at 6 weeks after flooding indicating slow release of N from organic manures (Deka Medhi *et al.*, 1996).

Blue Green Algae (BGA)

These are photosynthetic prokaryotic micro-organisms capable of fixing atmospheric nitrogen and found suitable under field condition. The predominant genera of N fixing BGA in 32 per cent of Indian rice soils are: (a) Anabaena, (b) Nostoc, (c) Aulosira, (d) Calothrix, and (e) Tolypothrix. In submerged rice field, BGA could add 20-30 kg N/ha during a season.

Azolla

It is a floating water fern having symbiotic relationship with N-fixing Cyanobacterium, *Anabaena azollae*. It produces 2-4 kg bio-mass/ha a day, incorporated 10 tonnes fresh matter per ha and contributes equivalent to 25-40 kg N/ha However, limitations in effective usage of Azolla are: (1) less water availability, (2) low survival rate during summer with

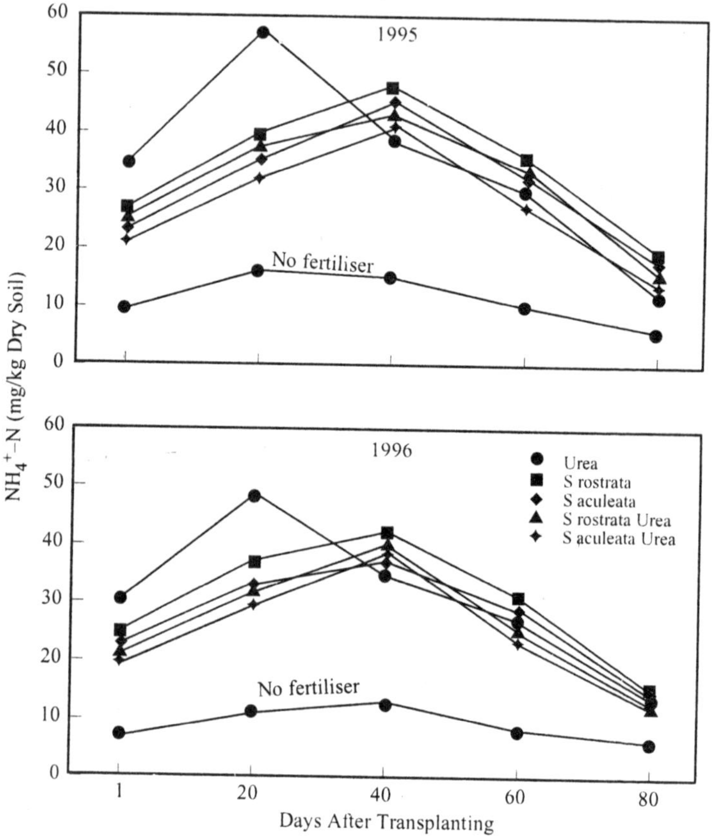

Fig. 5.1: Changes of Exchangeable NH_4^+–N (mg/kg dry soil) in soil as affected by Green Manures and Urea

temperature over 35-45°C, (3) high phosphate requirement of 60-80 kg/ha for good growth, (4) problem of transportation of 10-12 tonnes required for one ha rice, and (5) arthropods menace affecting the growth.

Organic Manures

This influence physical, chemical and micro-biological properties of soil and ultimately influence crop yield favourably. On an average, organic manures such as FYM and compost contain 0.5-1.0 per cent N, 0.6 per cent P_2O_5 and 0.5 per cent K_2O.

Phukan (1996) revealed that grain yield of sali rice was affected significantly due to incorporation of different organic manures

(Table 5.1). Maximum grain yields were recorded at 100 per cent N (Prilled urea) which was at par with 75 per cent N (PU) + 25 per cent N (Press-mud) and 75 per cent N (PU) + 25 per cent N (Rice straw). In another experiment at Regional Agricultural Research Station, Titabar, Bhattacharyya *et al.* (1995) revealed that substitution of inorganic N up to 50 per cent of the recommended level through application of FYM (10 t/ha) and rice straw (5 t/ha) could fetch higher addition produce over the control and recommended inorganic N.

Table 5.1: Yield of Transplanted Rice as Affected by Integrated Nutrient Management

Treatment	Grain Yield (q/ha)		
	1991	1992	Pooled
Control	29.27	27.32	28.29
100% N (PU)	42.30	38.81	40.55
75% N (PU) + 25% N (BS)	42.15	38.60	40.37
50% N (PU) + 50% N (BS)	39.72	37.09	38.40
25% N (PU) + 75% N (BS)	37.32	35.64	36.48
100% N (BS)	34.28	32.40	38.34
75% N (PU) + 25% N (PM)	41.40	38.41	39.90
50% N (PU) + 50% N (PM)	39.56	36.70	38.13
25% N (PU) + 75% N (PM)	37.12	34.85	35.98
100% N (PM)	33.74	32.00	32.87
75% N (PU) + 25% N (RS)	41.36	37.88	39.62
50% N (PU) + 50% N (RS)	38.64	36.56	37.60
25% N (PU) + 75% N (RS)	36.40	34.32	35.36
100% N (RS)	33.36	31.62	32.49
$CD_{(0.05)}$	1.13	0.93	0.76

PU = Prilled urea, BS = Bio-digested slurry, PM = Press-mud, RS = Rice straw.

Crop Residue Management

Crop residues include such materials as straw, stalks, husks, and leaves. In India, about 100 million tonnes of crop residues are available for recycling annually. The crop residues are a large reservoir of plant nutrients containing 0.5, 0.6 and 1.5 million tonnes of N, P_2O_5 and K_2O, respectively. Residues improve physical, chemical and biological properties also protect the soil from wind and water erosion. This is not only improves soil fertility but also increases crop yield. In rice growing areas, the most abundant and easily available organic manures are the rice straw and in due course, the rice husks. Ali *et al.* (1995) reported that incorporation of straw significantly influenced the grain yield of rice (Table 5.2). In an another experiment at Assam Agricultural

University, incorporation of rice and wheat straw in combination with N, P and K levels increased 1000 grain weight of rice significantly. Although grain yield of rice was non-significant, but there is an increasing trend (Anon., 1998).

Table 5.2: Effect of Rice Straw in Combination with Different Levels of Nitrogen, Phosphorus and Potassium Fertilisers

Treatment	Yield (q/ha)		Nutrient Uptake (kg/ha)		
	Grain	Straw	N	P	K
With rice straw	32.44	60.91	74.70	25.70	81.90
Without rice straw	28.29	54.41	54.41	61.30	70.00
$CD_{(0.05)}$	0.75	1.05	1.70	0.80	2.10
Levels of fertilisers (N : P : K :: 40 : 20 : 20 kg/ha)					
No NPK	25.50	48.70	53.10	16.80	60.50
50 per cent NPK	27.50	50.40	60.10	19.40	65.90
75 per cent NPK	30.40	65.60	66.20	22.50	74.10
100 per cent NPK	32.50	61.20	72.90	24.80	80.70
125 per cent NPK	32.70	64.00	77.30	27.90	85.40
150 per cent NPK	33.20	65.20	78.90	29.20	88.70
$CD_{(0.05)}$	1.30	1.80	3.00	1.40	3.40

The ability of soil to produce good and stable crop is dependent upon the physico-chemical condition of the soil. Ali *et al.* (1995) reported that organic manures led to an increase in action exchange capacity, organic matter and decreased bulk density. Available N, P and K also increased significantly (Table 5.3).

Green Manure

A large number of crops and plant species have been used as green manure to increase rice production (Table 5.4). Green manuring for the benefit of crops is an age old practice. In needs adequate attention at present as it is cheapest locally available resource for building up soil fertility and supplementing plant nutrients, especially nitrogen. In a field experiment, DekaMedhi and Medhi (1999) reported that addition of green manures and urea increased grain yield, straw yield and N uptake significantly from that of the control (Table 5.5). In an another experiment Sarma *et al.* (1997) and Anon. (1998) reported that grain and straw yield of rice significantly increased with the addition of organic manures alone and in combination with different levels of N, P

Table 5.3: Effect of Rice Straw and Fertiliser Levels on Some Physico-chemical Properties in Rice Soil

Treatment	pH (0-20 cm.)	CEC [cmol(p+)/kg] 0-20 cm.	Organic matter (g/kg)		Bulk density (g/cc)		Available N (kg/ha) 0—20 cm.	Available P (kg/ha) 0—20 cm.	Available K (kg/ha) 0—20 cm.
			0—20 cm.	20—40 cm.	0—20 cm.	20—40 cm.			
With rice straw	5.2	6.13	8.1	7.1	1.37	1.52	256.24	10.73	78.30
Without rice straw	5.2	6.10	7.1	6.6	1.47	1.58	253.15	10.03	74,50
$CD_{(0.05)}$	NS	NS	0.2	0.2	0.01	0.01	1.39	0.67	1.50
Levels of NPK fertilisers (N : P : K :: 40 : 20 : 20 kg/ha)									
No NPK	5.2	6.10	7.5	6.8	1.42	1.56	253.30	9.32	73.21
50 per cent NPK	5.2	6.11	7.7	6.9	1.42	1.54	254.97	9.95	75.46
75 per cent NPK	5.3	6.15	7.7	6.8	1.41	1.51	255.60	10.72	75.58
100 per cent NPK	5.2	6.11	7.6	6.8	1.42	1.55	254.71	10.50	76.66
125 per cent NPK	5.2	6.10	7.7	6.7	1.42	1.54	255.08	10.53	78.29
150 per cent NPK	5.3	6.11	7.7	6.9	1.42	1.57	255.70	11.24	79.70
$CD_{(0.05)}$	NS	NS	NS	NS	NS	NS	NS	1.15	2.61

Initial pH 5.2; CEC 6.1 cmol(p^+)/kg; Organic matter 7.1 g/kg; Bulk density 1.52 g/cc; Available N 256.59 kg/ha; Available P_2O_5 9.93 kg/ha; Available K_2O 73.35 kg/ha.

and K (Table 5.6). The highest grain and straw yields were obtained with the application of 50 per cent N, P, K + 10 t/ha FYM.

Table 5.4: Some Common Green Manure Crops

Local Name	Botanical Name	Growing Season	Green Manure Yield (t/ha)	N Content (%)
Sun hemp	*Crotolaria juncea*	Wet season	21.2	0.43
Dhaincha	*Sesbania aculeata*	Do	20.0	1.00
Rostrata	*Sesbania rostrata*	Do	30.0	2.50
Mung bean	*Phaseolus aureus*	Do	8.0	0.53
Cowpea	*Vigna sinensis*	Do	15.0	0.49
Senji	*Melilotus alba*	Dry season	26.6	0.57
Khesari	*Lathyrus sativa*	Do	12.3	0.54
Berseem	*Trifolium alexandrium*	Do	1.55	0.43

Table 5.5: Effect of Green Manure and Urea on Yield and N Nutrition of Rice (Mean over 2 years)

Treatment (40 kg N/ha)	Grain Yield (t/ha)	Straw Yield (t/ha)	N Uptake by Crop (kg/ha)
Control (No N)	2.8	3.3	21.10
Urea	5.4	4.3	47.72
Sesbania rostrata	5.6	4.2	45.74
Sesbania aculeata	4.7	4.1	39.38
S. rostrata (20 kg N/ha) + Urea (20 kg N/ha)	5.3	4.2	45.91
S. aculeata (20 kg N/ha) + Urea (20 kg N/ha)	4.9	4.2	43.92
$CD_{(0.05)}$	0.1	0.4	10.34

Most of the applied N was lost from the submerged rice field by different ways. Among these, ammonia volatilisation and leaching losses could be minimised with the incorporation of green manures and organic manures. Medhi *et al.* (1997) revealed that the cumulative loss of N was significantly lower due to incorporation of organic sources alone or in combination with urea than that of urea alone (Table 5.7). Ahmed *et al.* (1998) reported that incorporation of green manures and organic manures alone and in combination with urea decreased leaching loss of N than that of urea applied alone (Table 5.7).

Conclusion

Thus integrated nutrient management has shown greater potential in

Table 5.6: Integrated Effect of Chemical Fertilisers and Organic Manures on Yields of Rice

Treatment	Grain Yield (q/ha)				Straw Yield (q/ha)			
	1996	1997	1998	Mean	1996	1997	1998	Mean
No fertiliser NPK	32.71	26.62	24.55	27.96	40.83	57.71	58.53	52.35
100 per cent NPK (N : P : K :: 40 : 20 : 20 kg/ha)	48.55	29.12	30.46	36.04	54.86	61.15	68.38	61.46
75 per cent NPK + 5 t/ha FYM	44.17	33.37	34.31	37.28	53.05	65.94	72.23	63.74
75 per cent NPK + 5 t/ha pressmud	43.13	36.26	35.00	38.13	44.41	78.65	72.69	65.25
75 per cent NPK + 5 t/ha biogas slurry	46.25	32.79	35.20	38.08	49.44	72.00	77.37	66.27
75 per cent NPK + 5 t/ha *Sesbania rostrata*	46.25	30.47	35.18	37.30	47.77	76.19	73.41	65.79
50 per cent NPK + 10 t/ha FYM	49.25	35.30	35.61	40.05	58.19	69.53	70.71	66.14
50 per cent NPK + 10 t/ha pressmud	43.34	31.25	32.70	35.76	58.05	66.66	70.65	65.12
50 per cent NPK + 10 t/ha biogas slurry	45.00	35.87	32.98	37.95	53.33	71.93	69.67	64.97
50 per cent NPK + 10 t/ha *Sesbania rostrata*	47.71	31.44	34.10	37.75	45.55	70.24	72.59	62.79
$CD_{(0.05)}$	7.89	5.40	6.30	—	11.05	9.75	8.95	—

stabilising the yields of transplanted rice and also improves the soil physico-chemical properties.

Table 5.7: Cumulative Losses of Nitrogen through Ammonia Volatilisation and Leaching during 0-15 days as Affected by Different Sources of Nitrogen

Treatment (40 kg N/ha)	Cumulative Ammonia Loss				Cumulative Leaching Loss	
	1994		1995		1995	
	kg/ha	% of applied N	kg/ha	% of applied N	kg/ha	% of applied N loss
No fertiliser N	0.68	—	0.70	—	0.28	—
Urea	5.52	12.10	5.47	11.92	1.96	4.20
Farm yard manure	4.10	8.55	3.97	8.17	0.99	1.77
Sesbania rostrata	3.91	8.08	3.81	7.77	0.97	1.72
Sesbania aculeata	3.69	7.53	3.63	7.32	0.93	1.62
½ FYM + ½ urea	3.74	7.65	3.69	7.47	0.90	1.55
½ *S. rostrata* + ½ urea	3.55	7.18	3.49	6.97	0.86	1.45
½ *S. aculeata* + ½ urea	3.25	6.43	3.20	6.25	0.84	1.40
$CD_{(0.05)}$	0.87	2.67	0.83	2.64	0.34	0.67

Epilogue

1. Proper utility of legumes could be expanded suited to different situation to sustain the productivity of rice.
2. Efficient utilisation of organic waste, biofertilisation and easy adaptability by the farming community need to be explored.
3. Specific development of integrated nutrient system for rice and rice based systems in different ecosystem is needed.

REFERENCES

Ahmed, P.; Medhi, D.N. and DekaMedhi, B. (1998). "Influence of Organic Manures and Urea on Leaching Loss in Lowland rice Ecosystem", *J. Agric. Sci. Soc. NE India*, 11(1): 101-102.

Ali, A.; Medhi, D.N.; DekaMedhi, B. and Baroova, S.R. (1995). "Effect of Rice Straw and Fertilizer Levels on Some Physico-chemical Properties in Rice Soils", *J. Agric. Sci. Soc. NE India* 8(1): 131-32.

Ali, A.; Medhi, D.N.; DekaMedhi, B. and Baroova, S.R. (1995). "Effect of Rice Straw in Combination with Different Levels of Nitrogen, Phosphorus and Potash on Transplanted Rice", *J. Agric. Sci. Soc. NE India*, 8(2): 248-50.

Anon (1998). "Progress Report of Integrated Nutrient Management for Intensive Cropping System under High Rainfall Area", AAU, Jorhat-785013.

Bhattacharyya, H.C.; Saud, R.K. and Saikia, L. (1995). Partial Substitution of Inorganic Nitrogen through Organics in Kharif Rice. Proceedings of the National Seminar on "Problems and Prospects of Agriculture Development in N.E. India", November 27, 1995, *Agric. Sci. Soc. NE India*, Assam Agricultural University, Jorhat-785013.

DekaMedhi, B.; Barthakur, H.P. and Barthakur, S.N. (1966). "Effect of Organic and Inorganic Source of Nitrogen on the Nutrients in Soil and Soil Solution and Growth of Rice", *J. Indian Soc. Sci*, 44: 263-66.

DekaMedhi, B. and Medhi, D.N. (1999). "Effect of Green Manures and Urea on Nitrogen Mineralization in Relation to Growth of Rice under Upper Brahmaputra Valley Zone of Assam", *Indian J. Agric. Sci.*, 69(3): In Press.

Medhi, D.N.; Ahmed, P.; DekaMedhi, B.; Baroova, S.R. and Sarma, A.C. (1977). Influence of Green Manures and Urea on Ammonia Volatilization Loss and Yield of Transplanted Rice, Proceedings of the International Symposium on "Rainfed Rice Production Strategy for 21st Century", November 25-27, 1997, Assam Agricultural University, Jorhat-785013.

Phukan, D. (1996). Unpublished Ph.D. thesis, "Integrated Nutrient Management in Summer Rice-Winter Rice Cropping Sequence", Assam Agricultural University, Jorhat-785013.

Prasad, R. and De Datta, S.K. (1979). "Increasing Fertilizer Nitrogen Efficiency in Wetland Rice", 465-84, *In*: Nitrogen and Rice, Institute Rice Research Institute, P.O. Box 933, Manila, Philippines.

Sarma, A.C.; Medhi, D.N.; DekaMedhi, B. and Thakur, A.C. (1997). Integrated Nutrient Management on Rice-linseed Cropping Sequence in High Rainfall Areas. Proceedings of the International Symposium on "Rainfed Rice Production Strategy for 21st Century", November 25-27, 1997, Assam Agriculture University, Jorhat-785013.

6

INTEGRATED NUTRIENT MANAGEMENT IN DIRECT SEEDED RICE

— *H.C. Bhattacharyya*

The world population will grow to 7.2 billion up from the 5.3 billion of 1990 leaving 200 million in South Asia under-nourished by 2010 A.D. The continuous pressure on lands for non-agricultural uses including human settlements, will make land scarcities very acute. Since the frontiers of arable land are almost closed in most of countries, future increases in agricultural production to meet a demand expanding at a high annual rate, must occur primarily through increases in yield per unit area per unit time.

About 30 million sq. km. of land or over 30 per cent of the world's exploitable soils are under upland and shifting cultivation, where rice is the principal food crop, producing the bulk of the food for nearly 10 per cent of the world population. Rice is mostly direct seeded or dibbled under rainfed conditions in such areas having wide variations with respect to their natural fertility physical properties, topography and cropping patterns. The agriculture in such areas is of subsistence type with very small size of holding and very poor yield due to fragile eco-system, uncertain water availability, land erodability, poor nutrient status and soil acidity. In shifting cultivation, the soil becomes fragile after 2-3 years of cropping. Because of the population pressure, the fallow period in shifting cultivation is shortened increasing the cropping period, resulting in failure to restore soil fertility, which is a threat to sustainable agriculture. Integrated nutrient management, therefore, holds the key for restoring soil health over and above improving crop productivity.

Direct Seeded Rice

Direct seeded rice is a very common system of rice culture in uplands, lowlands and in deep water rice areas. The practice eliminates nursery raising and transplanting and thereby saves time, energy and money. In the uplands, deep water situations, under shifting cultivation of the North East India and as a rainfed summer crop in lowlands direct seeded rice culture is a routine method of rice cultivation. This culture covers almost one-forth to one-fifth of rice areas of the region. The cropping pattern in uplands are found crop based, particularly rice, maize and root crops like cassava, grown either as a mixed, sequential, inter or relay crop according to farmers' need, land type water availability and market availability. The yields are very poor due to small and fragmented holding, subsistence farming, fragile ecosystem, land erodability, poor nutrient status and soil acidity.

Advantages of Direct Seeded Rice

* Lower labour requirement.
* Eliminates seedling raising, uprooting and transplanting.
* Less water requirement.
* Matures 7-10 days earlier than transplanting.
* Sowing in dry soil before monsoon is possible.

Disadvantages of Direct Seeding

* Poor establishment and plant stand.
* High weed infestation.
* Low tillering.
* Tendency to lodge due to poor root development.

Most of the direct seeded rice areas have poor soil with uncertain rainfall distribution and are grown by the poorest of the poors using traditional methods with low or no inputs, either under permanent or shifting cultivation. With high anticipated population growth the productivity of rice will have to be raised using organic/green manures or biofertilisers requiring least investment.

Resource Use in Direct Seeded Rice Growing Area

Traditional cropping systems are highly complex and diverse because the farmers attempt to achieve their multiple objectives simultaneously. The traditional low input direct seeded system though fetch low productivity, is never risk prone. The system of mixed, relay and intercropping, conserve soil, restore fertility enhances biological water harvest and utilisation and maintain ecosustainability through minimum tillage, low or no chemical use and use of native fertility. These are accomplished through the use of indigenous knowledge of farmers which are culture and locality bound, fragmentary, multidimensional and experimental *in situ*. Alley cropping, in which tree biomss is used to cover and protect the soil in addition to soil nitrogen recycling, is prevalent in hill farming. Contour hedge rows with trees is also practiced in the same line.

Most of the present systems, are, however, un-scientific and not systematised, while the concept should be to decrease environmental degradation and preserve natural resources for ecologically stable farming which is self-sustaining with low input, diversification and productiveness. For a system to be stable, it must maintain or improve soil structure, prevent accelerated soil erosion, preserve or improve soil organic matter land have a built-in nutrient recycling mechanism.

As better yielding materials and fertilisers are available, as legume seeds inoculated with highly active N_2 fixing bacteria becomes widely used, yields will be raised and extension of cropping periods in shifting cultivation will have less and less detrimental effect besides meeting the diverse needs of farmers.

Integrated Nutrient Management

Because of high cost of chemical fertilisers, integrated soil fertility management that can better recycle native and applied nutrients and incorporate biologically fixed nitrogen, need to be promoted especially in poor soil conditions where direct seeded rice is grown. The increase in organic component in the soil results in reduced leaching, reducing of toxic level of aluminium and improvement of soil health.

The role of biomas addition in relation to nutrition of the direct seeded rice was evaluated at IARI and it was found that addition of *Dhaincha* (*Seshania* sp.) and *Subabul*, as green manure with 50 per cent of the recommended fertiliser dose gave as high yield as from the full dose (100-50-50). Green manure added 50-60 kg N/ha to the soil for succeeding crop of rice (Table 6.1). State farming, however, did not gave a consistent result because of variability in the weed population.

It has been reported that organic manure should be applied at the time of land preparation at the rate of 5 to 10 t/ha along with 60 kg N, 40 kg P_2O_5 and 20 kg K_2O per ha for tall varieties (Prasad *et al.*, 1986). For the direct seeded rice crop, one-fourth N, 15 days after seeding, half N at maximum tillering and the rest one-fourth N at visual panicle initiation will be useful. For mechanised sowing (drill) basal application of N and P_2O_5 may be done at least 10 cm below the soil surface. To increase the fertiliser use efficiency as well as water use efficiency, adequate quantity of organic be applied along with inorganic fertilisers as basal dose, especially where green manuring or feeder-*cum*-green manuring with legumes has not been followed which will greatly improve yield through stabilisation of pH, supplying organic matter and N, serving as a slow N releasing compound, as well as minimising the toxic effects of salts (Anonymous, 1983).

Table 6.1: Integrated Nutrient Management in Direct Seeded Rice

Nutrient Management	Grain Yield (g/ha)		
	1984	1985	1986
Full fertiliser (100-50-50 kg N-P-K/ha)	36.6	47.0	34.1
Half fertiliser	27.1	33.1	26.9
Half fertiliser + *dhaincha*	39.4	52.0	36.7
Half fertiliser + *Subabul*	37.6	52.0	32.2
Half fertiliser + State farming	31.0	49.8	35.1
CD (0.05)	1.2	1.7	1.4

Source: Singh, Mishra and Bhattacharyya (1987).

Experiments conducted at different locations showed that (Table 6.2) irrespective of levels, 25 per cent of N could be substituted with FYM without adverse effect on yield. Even in some locations FYM could replace as much as 50 per cent of N requirement, while in some other (Masodha) FYM was not found to be advantageous in respect of yield.

Table 6.2: Yield (Q/ha) of Rice at Different Manurial Sources

Centre	100% N (Chemical)	75% N (Chem) + 25% N (FYM)	50% N (Chem) + 50% N (FYM)	Whole N (FYM)	CD (0.05)
R.S. Pura	39.8	38.7	37.8	34.5	2.98
Masodha	34.6	32.4	29.8	25.8	1.38
Pusa farm	29.4	27.7	24.9	20.6	2.62
Kapurthalla	37.8	38.0	36.0	29.4	2.15
Parbhani	12.9	12.9	13.1	11.9	0.82

Studies conducted at RARS, Titabar for 5 years also proved that use of FYM and rice straw before the rice crop not only increases rice yields but also reduces cost of cultivation, land increases net return (Table 6.3).

Table 6.3: Effect of Combination of Organic and Inorganic Nutrient Sources on Rice Yields over Five Years

Treatments	Addl. Produce Over Control	Addl. Income Over Control	Net Return (Rs.)
Control (No N)	—	—	—
Recommended N : P_2O_5 : K_2O (@ 30 : 20 : 20 kg/ha)	17.39	8,695.00	8,375.00
Green manuring (3 t/ha) + 50% N + P + K	17.37	8,685.00	8,585.00
Green manuring (3t/ha) + 25% N + P + K	15.30	7,650.00	7,570.00
FYM (10 t/ha) + 25% N + P + K	18.52	9,260.00	9,100.00
FYM (10 t/ha) + 25% N + P + K	15.34	7,670.00	7,590.00
Rice straw (5 t/ha) + 50% N + P + K	18.64	9,320.00	9,160.00
Rice straw (5 t/ha) + 25% N + P + K	15.93	7,965.00	7,855.00

Rice direct needed in aerobic soils is exposed to many adverse conditions not found under flooded conditions. On strongly acid soils soluble aluminium and manganese may reach levels toxic to the rice plant. Incorporation of organics like FYM, compost, green manure, increases pH value of soils and reduces aluminium toxicity. Leguminous weeds and tree species available in the surroundings can effectively be utilised.

Increasing cropping intensity and residue incorporation in the soil, is also one of the component of integrated nutrient management practices. The rape-rice-soybean system has been found to accumulate highest organic matter in the soil. The importance of returning all crop residues has been emphasised globally time and again (McCollum *et al.*, 1987, McIntesh *et al.*, 1981). The continuous application of rice straw increases organic matter and CEC, has been established by various workers. The biomas produced by legumes in the system, help to build up the soil organic matter when incorporated. In Entisol, blackgram-rice system is known to increase the organic carbon balance (George and Prasad, 1989). In the red soils alley cropping with *Subabul,* as hedge row crop increases organic carbon and pH of the soil (Soepardi, 1989). Appropriate cover crops in the rice-fallow system with legumes not only reduces soil erosion but also improves infiltration (Lal, 1984). Rice-must-Summer pulse system may be the most useful, diverse and remunerative systems in north east India. In parts if Eastern India direct seeded rice-horsegram/ chick pea/rapeseed/linseed are common. Monocropping of rice, rice-rice-pulses, rice-finger millet-pulses and rice-sweet potato are the feasible cropping systems in Tripura.

Table 6.4: Grain Yield (t/ha) of Rice in Sequential Cropping with Food Legumes

Treatment	Mean of 3 years	
	No Urea N	100 kg Urea N
Bare fallow after rice	1.3	5.3
Soybean residue returned	2.0	5.4
Green gram—residue returned	1.4	5.0
Sesbania—residue returned	2.3	5.7
Sorghum/rice—straw returned	1.2	4.9

Source: Chapman and Myers (1987).

Tropical feed legumes nodulates effectively with cowpea type rhizobea which are widely distributed in the tropics. Since farmers look for multiple benefits for their investments, legumes may provide multiple use solutions to be acceptable (Table 6.4). Short duration pulses such as mungbean and cowpea, offer an attractive benefit of grains for human consumption and residues for green manuring. Studies at IRRI revealed that food-forage legume systems can increase cereal yield, produce legume grain crops and forage legumes especially during dry season when animal feed is limited, decreases the use of fertilisers and increases the total fodder available to animals in the small farms. The attractive feature of utilising legumes in cropping systems is that they usually do not compete for resources with the associated crop.

Recommendations

Following recommendations emerged from the Seminar on "Integrated Plant Nutrient Supply Systems" with special reference to NEU Region:

1. In Integrated Unit Nutrient Supply System efforts are to be initiated on the following lines:

   (a) Increase the consumption of Chemical Fertiliser by 30-40 per cent.

   (b) Efforts should be made to maintain N-P-K ratio.

   (c) Chemical fertiliser should be invariably supplemented

with organic manures, biofertilisers and neem products to prevent N losses.

2. Sale of Chemical Fertiliser should be encouraged through private trade and small dealers (10 tonnes stock) should be expempted from licensing.
3. Stress should be given to increase the Chemical Fertiliser in fruit plants to an optimum level of 70 kg (N-P-K) in a ratio 0.75 : 0.50 : 1.0.
4. Agriculture Universities and Research Organisations like ICAR and others should take up R&D works on biofertilisers on priority basis.

REFERENCES

1. Anonymous (1983). *Final Planning Report Kifil Shinafiya Project*, Vol. 7, Rice Cultivation, Water and Power Consultancy Service (India) Ltd., New Delhi.
2. Bhattacharyya, H.C., Saud, R.K. and Saikia, L. (1995). *Partial Substitution of Inorganic Nitrogen through Organics in Kharif Rice*, Proc. Sem. Agric. Sci. Soc. NE India, Nov. 27-28, 1995, 199-23.
3. Chapman, A.L. and Myers, R.J.K. (1987). "Nitrogen Contributed by Grain Legumes in Rotation with Rice on the Cununurra Soils of the Ord. Irrigated Area," *Australian J. Exptl. Agricultural*, 27, 155-63.
4. George, M. and Prasad, R. (1989). "Studies on the Effect of Cereal-Cereal and Cereal-Legume Cropping Systems on the Productivity and Fertility of Soil," *Fertiliser News*, 34(5), 21-25.
5. Lal, R. (1984). "Land Management—Management of Soil Physical Properties for Soil and Water Conservation and Seed Bed Preperation in West Africa," in *An Overview of Upland Rice Research*, pp. 383-94, IRRI, Los Banos, Philippines.
6. McCollum, R.E., Arevalo, L. and Aznaran, A. (1987). "Phosphorus, Zinc and Copper Fertilisation," in *Tropical Soils—Tech. Report, 1985-86* (N. Caude and McCants, eds.), pp. 57-88, North Carolina State University, Roleigh, North Carolina.
7. McIntosh, J.L., Ismail, I.G., Effendi, S. and Sudjadi, M. (1981). "Cropping Systems to Preserve Fertility of Red Yellow Podzolic Soils of Indonesia", *Int. Symp. on Distribution, Characterization and Utilization of Problem Soils*, pp. 409-29, Trop. Agric. Res. Centre, Tsukuba, Japan.
8. Prasad, R.B., Tomar, J.B. and Singh, N.P. (1986). "Direct Seeded Rice", *Indian Fmg.*, 36(2) : 28-29.
9. Singh, K.N., Mishra, B.N. and Bhattacharyya, H.C. (1987). "Direct Seeded Rice—A Viable Alternative for Transplanted Rice", Paper presented in *the Nat. Symp. on Alternate Farming Systems*, I.S.A., Feb. 21-23, New Delhi.
10. Soepardi, G. (1989). "Nitrogen and Other Nutrient in Red Yellow Podzolics of Kumai, Central Kalimatin under Alley Cropping Systems", in *Nutrient Management for Food Crop Production in Tropical Farming Systems*, pp. 177-85.

7

AGRICULTURAL PRODUCTION AND FERTILISER CONSUMPTION WITH SPECIAL REFERENCE TO NORTH EAST AREA

— *L. Joshi*

Out of 329 million hectares geographical area, the country is having 181 million hectares of agricultural land. The major crops are Wheat and Rice which occupy about 42 and 24 million hectares. The total area of agricultural land is split into 97.16 million holdings leading to small average holdings size of 1.7 hectares.

The country's population is growing very fast. To feed the additional population the foodgrain production has to be increased at a faster rate. To increase foodgrain production the fertiliser plays an important role. The consumption of fertilisers N-P-K in 1997-98 was 16,195 thousand mt. with a per hectare consumption of 86 kg plant nutrient at a ratio of 7.9 : 2.9 : 1. The production of N & P in the country is 10,083 thousand mts. N and 3058.3 mt. P_2O_5 respectively during 1997-98. Foodgrain production during 1997-98 was 193 million mts. Expected foodgrain production during 1998-99 is about 202 million mt.

The country has become almost self-sufficient so far urea production is concerned. However, the country has to depend 100 per cent on import for potassic fertiliser and about 25 per cent for phosphatic fertiliser. The year-wise consumption of fertilisers (N-P-K) in India for different years and N-P-K ratio are given in Table 7.1.

After decontrol of Phosphatic and Potassic fertilisers, the consumption of these fertilisers reduced drastically during 1992-93. To maintain the proper N-P-K ratio and to retain sustainable agriculture, the Government of India decided to give ad hoc concession on phosphatic and potassic fertilisers to make the price affordable to farmers. However, the policy of ad hoc concession is not consistent.

Table 7.1: All-India Consumption of N, P_2O_5 and K_2O and N-P-K Ratio

('000 mts.)

Year	N	P_2O_5	K_2O	Total	N-P-K Ratio
1950-51	55	9	6	70	9.2 : 1.5 :1
1955-56	108	13	10	131	10.4 : 1.3 : 1
1960-61	212	53	29	294	7.3 : 1.8 : 1
1965-66	575	133	77	785	7.4 : 1.7 : 1
1970-71	1,479	541	236	2,257	6.3 : 2.3 : 1
1975-76	2,149	467	278	2,894	7.7 : 1.7 : 1
1980-81	3,678	1,214	624	5,516	5.9 : 1.9 : 1
1985-86	5,661	2,005	808	8,474	7.0 : 2.5 : 1
1990-91	7,997	3,221	1,328	12,546	6.0 : 2.4 : 1
1991-92	8,046	3,321	1,361	12,728	5.9 : 2.4 : 1
1992-93	8,427	2,844	884	12,155	9.5 : 3.2 : 1
1993-94	8,789	2,669	908	12,366	9.7 : 2.9 : 1
1994-95	9,507	2,932	1,124	13,563	8.5 : 2.6 : 1
1995-96	9,823	2,897	1,156	13,876	8.4 : 2.5 : 1
1996-97	13,302	2,976	1,030	14,308	10.0 : 2.9 : 1
1997-98	10,905	3,917	1,373	16,195	7.9 : 2.9 : 1

At present, the Government of India is allowing Rs. 4,400 concession on indigenous DAP, Rs. 3,000 on imported DAP, Rs. 3,000 on Potash, Rs. 900 on SSP and Rs. 3,000-4,000 on different complex fertilisers. Urea is the only controlled fertiliser at the moment, and is under retention price scheme (RPS).

North East Region

North-Eastern region comprising of the states of Assam, Manipur, Nagaland, Meghalaya, Tripura, Arunachal Pradesh and Mizoram is predominantly hilly in nature. The topography is mountainous except Assam valley. The climate varies from sub-tropical to temperate. Monsoon is the principal rainy season in this region accounting for 65 per cent of total rainfall.

This region has relatively more share in the country with regard to the natural resources of land (7.75%), forests (15.29%) and water (11% of total precipitation in the country). However, it contributes to only 2.98 per cent to the net national domestic product. The economy of this region is mainly dependent on agriculture, which is subsistence in nature.

North-eastern soils fall under the order of Ultlsols, Oxisols, Alfisols, Inceptisols, Mollisols and Entisols. These soils are generally rich in unhumified organic matter, medium to high in available nitrogen, low in available phosphorous, low to high is available in potash and low available B and MO. Soil erosion and acidity are the important soil problem in this region.

Consumption in North East

The NPK consumption ratios in North East shows a slightly different picture from the All-India average. The NPK ratio in Meghalaya (27.6 : 12.6 : 1) and Manipur (18.7 : 2.5 : 1) shows a significant imbalance in favour of Nitrogen, the other states are Arunachal Pradesh, Assam, Mizoram, Nagaland and Tripura do not seem to exhibit this trend. However, the Tea Board in North East shows a very high imbalance in favour of both Nitrogen and Phosphorous ratio. Fertiliser consumption (N-P-K) of North-Eastern region and N-P-K ratio as given in Tables 7.2 and 7.3.

Table 7.2: Statewise Consumption of Plant Nutrients per Unit of Cropped Area 1996-97 and 1997-98

State	1996-97				1997-98			
	N	P_2O_5	K_2O	Total	N	P_2O_5	K_2O	Total
East	42.1	11.4	7.1	60.6	43.7	14.9	8.4	67.0
Assam	8.4	1.5	4.7	14.6	10.0	3.9	4.6	18.6
Arunachal Pradesh	1.3	0.5	0.4	2.2	1.3	0.5	0.4	2.2
Manipur	42.0	4.6	2.0	48.6	40.7	5.5	2.2	48.3
Meghalaya	9.2	4.4	0.8	14.4	9.3	4.2	0.3	13.9
Mizoram	2.1	0.9	0.5	3.5	1.8	3.9	2.9	8.7
Nagaland	1.9	1.6	0.4	3.8	1.3	1.1	0.3	2.6
Sikkim	4.3	1.4	0.2	5.9	3.8	2.2	0.6	6.5
Tripura	11.8	4.1	2.9	18.8	13.8	5.0	3.8	22.7

Due to relatively low yield of foodgrain crops and higher availability of organic manures per hectare cultivated area compared to the country, the deficiency of micro-nutrients in these states has not been felt to the same extent as in some other states. However, these deficiencies are likely to aggravate with more area coming under High Yield Variety crops and more concerted efforts to raise productivity through use of enhanced doses of fertilisers.

The productivity of foodgrain crops has commensurated with the application of fertiliser nutrients in various states of the region. Manipur and Tripura where per hectare application of N, P and K is higher, productivity of foodgrains is also higher than other states in the region.

Table 7.3: Statewise Consumption Ratio of N, P_2O_5 and K_2O during 1996-97 and 1997-98

States	1996-97			1997-98		
	N	P_2O_5	K_2O	N	P_2O_5	K_2O
East	6.0	1.6	1	5.2	1.8	1
Assam	1.8	0.3	1	2.2	0.8	1
Arunachal Pradesh	3.2	1.3	1	3.7	1.4	1
Manipur	21.1	2.3	1	18.7	2.5	1
Meghalaya	12.2	5.8	1	27.6	12.6	1
Mizoram	3.8	1.7	1	0.6	1.3	1
Nagaland	4.6	3.9	1	4.7	4.0	1
Sikkim	27.5	9.0	1	6.9	4.0	1
Tea Board	2,564.0	637.0	1	—	—	—
Tripura	4.1	1.4	1	3.6	1.3	1

The fertiliser nutrients response potential is only 16.4 per cent showing that there is a scope for improving yield in this region through adequate and judicious use of chemical fertilisers. The consumption of fertilisers is over all very low in the North East. There is a great scope to intensify use of fertilisers based on the nutrient consumption in North East. The gross cropped area, irrigated area, area under foodgrain and cropping intensity for the North East is given in Tables 7.4 and 7.5.

Analysis of the Situation in North East

In North East, shifting cultivation is predominant with an unique land tenure system, flood hazards, free range grazing, lack of proper communication, finance, suitable farming systems, low use of nutrients and marketing facilities are major constraints for the progress of this region.

(i) *Shifting Cultivation:* This is the foremost constraint in this area. It is practised all over the region covering the annual area of 3,86,500 hectares. This practice is uneconomical and leads to an annual loss of 88.3 million tonnes of soil and 10.67, 0.37 and 6.05 tonnes of N, P and K respectively. The cultivators desert the land once, the fertility of the soil is lost.

Table 7.4: Consumption of N, P_2O_5 and K_2O in Eastern and North-Eastern States during 1995-96 to 1997-98

('000 MT.)

State	1995-96				1996-97				1997-98			
	N	P_2O_5	K_2O	Total	N	P_2O_5	K_2O	Total	N	P_2O_5	K_2O	Total
Arunachal Pradesh	0.20	0.11	0.07	0.38	0.32	0.13	0.10	0.55	0.33	0.13	0.09	0.55
Assam	23.66	5.46	20.02	49.14	32.15	5.84	17.82	55.81	38.42	15.07	17.76	71.25
Manipur	10.54	1.05	0.24	11.83	11.39	1.25	0.54	13.18	11.02	1.48	0.59	13.09
Meghalaya	1.83	0.86	0.10	2.79	2.20	1.05	0.18	3.43	2.21	1.01	0.08	3.30
Mizoram	0.22	0.33	0.22	0.78	0.23	0.10	0.06	0.39	0.20	0.44	0.33	0.97
Nagaland	0.28	0.19	0.05	0.52	0.41	0.35	0.09	0.85	0.28	0.24	0.06	0.58
Sikkim	0.66	0.39	—	1.05	0.55	0.18	0.02	0.75	0.48	0.28	0.07	0.83
Tripura	5.33	1.58	1.54	8.45	5.41	1.88	1.33	8.62	6.35	2.31	1.76	10.42
Tea Board	25.94	5.72	0.04	31.70	25.64	6.37	0.01	32.02	30.30	8.70	—	39.00
West Bengal	512.20	195.22	140.30	847.72	528.17	224.56	143.37	896.10	546.62	259.86	169.63	976.11
Orissa	174.77	35.10	27.66	237.53	178.43	43.13	29.21	250.77	195.83	55.52	39.48	290.83
Bihar	558.17	117.87	44.01	720 05	639.21	100.65	45.97	785.83	645.19	159.41	55.87	860.47
Total	1,313.81	363.88	234.26	1,911.94	1,424.11	385.49	238.70	2,048.30	1,477.24	504.45	285.72	2,267.41

Table 7.5: Gross Cropped and Irrigated Area and Area under Foodgrains with Cropping Intensity (1994-95)

Zone/State	Cumulative Area		Cropping Intensity	Irrigated Area	Percen-tage	Area '000 Hectares	
	Net	Gross		Net	(5/2)	Area under Foodgrains	Percen-tage (7/3)
(1)	(2)	(3)	(4)	(5)	(6)	(7)	(8)
Arunachal Pradesh	140	252	168	36	24	178	71
Assam	2,777	3,825	138	572	21	2,668	70
Manipur	226	271	120	65	29	163	60
Meghalaya	201	238	118	45	22	130	55
Nagaland	206	221	107	62	30	187	85
Sikkim	95	127	134	16	17	77	61
Tripura	277	459	166	35	13	271	59
Mizoram	65	112	172	8	12	80	71
Total (NE)	3,999	5,505	1,123	839	21	3,754	67
Total (All-India)	142,819	188,147	132	62,909	37	123,860	66
Share of India	0.03	0.03	8.51	0.01	1	0.03	100.07

(ii) *Land Tenure System:* There is no permanent proprietary ownership right of the farmers over the land. They do not feel sense of belonging and do not invest on inputs for higher productivity.

(iii) Lack of suitable, economically viable and acceptable farming/cropping system.

(iv) Leaching of nutrients due to high rainfall.

(v) Lack of finance with the farmers leads to low purchase of inputs like seed, fertilisers and chemicals.

(vi) Low adaptability for new farming technology.

(vii) Inadequate infrastructure like road, market facilities.

(viii) Lack of communication, not getting fertilisers in time due to not having local factories.

(ix) Weak extension programmes leading to poor education to the farmers and high cost of transportation.

Remedial Measures

Considering the constraints for development of agriculture as well as increase in fertiliser consumption, it is necessary to look into the remedial measures for North East region which are given as below:

(i) Improving infrastructure facility and enhancing incentives to manufacturers/marketors to supply adequate quantity of fertiliser in these states.

(ii) Procurement of fertilisers with need based approach by the states and easy availability to the farmers.

(iii) To create awareness among the farmers about balanced use of nutrients.

(iv) Sil conservation measures are to be popularised among the farmers on slopy lands to reduce soil and nutrient loss due to soil erosion.

(v) Contour bunding is recommended since terracing is not financially feasible to the farmers.

(vi) Additional transport facility is to be provided in the extreme areas.

(vii) The farmer education programmes and extension programmes are to be extensively undertaken by the Government as well as fertiliser companies and voluntary organisations (NGOs).

(viii) Agro based industries are to be established considering the local need.

8

SOIL TESTING AND FERTILISER RECOMMENDATION

— S.K. Saha

The importance of fertilisers in increasing the production of foodgrains and other crops is being well recognised by the farmers with the advent of Green Revolution. Estimates by the World Bank for a 20-year period (1951-52 to 1972-73) reveal that the percentage of total yield increase due to fertiliser is of the order of 49 per cent. On the other hand, the importance of soil testing is aptly stated as "soil testing is to the art of crop production what the thermometer is to the medical profession". Soil testing and soil fertility management for sustainable crop production is, therefore, of great importance to any country. Soil testing is well recognised as a useful tool in making balanced and efficient use of fertilisers. Soil testing is a crucial service for advising farmers on fertiliser use. It enables a useful judgement on the plant-available nutrients present in the soil so that the balanced requirements can be supplied timely.

The great Soil Scientist Dr. J.S. Kanwar in 1971 said "We have come to a point where it is well understood that a misleading value is worse than no value at all, as fertiliser bill represents the heaviest item of expenditure for the farmer, particularly in developing countries like India".

A properly interpreted soil test provides the best means to estimate nutrient availability in the soil of a particular field.

Operationally, a soil fertility evaluation service programme begins and ends on the farm. The final recommendation received by the farmer can be no better than the information obtained from him and the quality of the soil sample taken from his field. The following information is required concerning:

— name of farmer
— full address of the farmer
— exact location of field
— irrigation frequency, adequacy, source
— drainage
— soil type
— previous cropping history and yields
— previous manuring history
— date of sampling
— slope
— salinity
— size of area represented by sample
— crop and variety to be grown during the season
— cropping pattern to be followed during next two years
— other relevant information available.

Soil samples from fields are generally collected by the staff members of State Department of Agriculture or field staff of fertiliser companies. Only a few number of soil samples are given directly by farmers reflecting on little enthusiasm amongst farmers.

One has to ensure obtaining good sample. The soil sample collected should be representative of the area sampled. A field can be treated as a single sampling unit only if it is appreciably uniform in all respects. The greatest source of error is usually the soil sample itself. The soil samples should be taken in a zig-zag pattern. A representative composite soil sample can be composed of 8 to 20 sub-samples from a uniform field. A common error in soil sampling occurs when the top few cm of soil are dry and not included in the normal sample.

The test methods generally adopted in the soil testing laboratories in India are given in Table 8.1.

Table 8.1: Soil Test Methods Used in India (Nutrient and Method Used)

Nitrogen	Phosphorus	Potassium
1. Organic Carbon (%)	1. Olsen's—P	1. Ammonium acetate—K
2. $KMnO_4$—N	2. Bray's—P	2. HNO_3—K
3. NO_3—N	3. Morgan's—P	
4. NH_4—N	4. Truog's—P	
5. $Ca(OH)_2$—N	5. North Carolina	

Interpretation of Soil Test Values

The numerical values derived from the chemical tests are usually interpreted into categories. This gives the results meaning so that fertiliser recommendations can be derived. In other words, converting a soil test values differently. This is partly due to difference in soils, climate and crops. It is also partly due to differences in fertiliser recommendation philosophies.

In India, the vital role of the soil-testing service in the development of agriculture through balanced fertilisation was recognised in the early 1950s with the establishment of 16 soil-testing laboratories under a joint Indo-American operational agreement for "Determination of Soil Fertility and Fertiliser Use". During last four and half decades, the soil testing service has significantly been grown, both in its content and size.

Soil Testing Laboratories and Their Analysing Capacity (1994-95)

At present, Soil Testing is provided through 497 number of Soil Testing Laboratories (run by State Government and Industries). These labs are spread over all the States and Union Territories of Chandigarh and Daman and Diu. Fertiliser Industries have established 65 number of Soil Testing Laboratories (33 Static and 32 Mobile in different States. Zone-wise number of soil testing labs. with their annual analysing capacity and % utilisation is given Tables 8.2 and 8.3.

Table 8.2: Details of State Soil Testing Laboratories in India

State	No. of Labs.			Analysing Capacity '000	% Utilisation 1994-95	No. of Sample Analysed Period ending Sept. 95
	S	M	Total			
(1)	(2)	(3)	(4)	(5)	(6)	(7)
South Zone						
Andhra Pradesh	23	4	27	338.0	94.00	—
Karnataka	19	3	22	608.0	112.80	—
Kerala	13	7	20	272.0	63.32	—
Tamil Nadu	14	15	29	1,000.0	116.20	—
Pondicherry	2	—	2	20.0	96.23	9,140
Andaman & Nicobar Islands	1	—	1	12.0	53.23	2,110
Total	72	29	101	2,250.0	105.28	1,1250

(Contd.)

Table 8.2: (*Contd.*)

(1)	(2)	(3)	(4)	(5)	(6)	(7)
West Zone						
Gujarat	14	7	21	210.0	94.53	17,135
Madhya Pradesh	19	5	24	360.0	41.22	
Rajasthan	8	12	20	248.0	87.00	95,274
Maharashtra	17	—	17	170.0	109.53	83,795
Goa	2	—	2	18.0	89.94	5,215
Dadra & Nagar Haveli	1	—	1	1.0	105.50	568
Total	61	24	85	1,007.0	76.10	2,01,987
North Zone						
Haryana	24	0	24	266.0	78.86	—
Punjab	43	9	52	515.0	83.35	2,43,142
Himachal Pradesh	11	—	11	70.0	75.07	22,692
Uttar Pradesh	56	15	71	440.0	105.57	2,36,052
Jammu & Kashmir	3	3	6	38.5	92.71	19,327
Delhi	1	—	1	5.0	115.74	1,468
Total	138	27	165	1,334.5	89.78	5,22,681
East Zone						
Bihar	32	—	32	310.0	15.33	—
Orissa	11	1	12	225.0	74.15	—
West Bengal	10	4	14	116.0	30.49	17,635
North East Zone						
Assam	7	4	11	102.51	67.31	41,522
Tripura	2	1	3	15.0	64.86	3,013
Manipur	1	0	1	10.0	—	1,067
Nagaland	1	0	1	20.0	8.0	—
Meghalaya	3	0	3	17.0	—	—
Arunachal Pradesh	1	—	1	5.0	21.43	—
Sikkim	1	1	2	13.0	102.89	6,475
Mizoram	1	—	1	8.0	—	2,405
Total	17	6	23	190.51	49.35	54,482
State Total	341	91	432	5,433.01	86.46	8,08,035
Soil Testing Labs with Fertiliser Ind.	33	32	65	603.5	54.63	1,72,664
Grand Total	374	123	497	6,036.51	83.23	9,80,699

Table 8.3: Details of Soil Testing Laboratories (Fertiliser Industry-wise) 1994-95

S.No.	Name of the Industry	No. of Labs.			Capacity '000	% Utilisation
		S	M	Total		
1.	Hindustan Fert. Cropn. Ltd.	12	13	25	190.00	6.10
2.	IFFCO	2	2	4	60.00	128.85
3.	Gujarat State Fert. Cropn. Ltd.	1	2	3	30.00	138.94
4.	Indian Potash Ltd.	—	3	3	30.00	37.84
5.	Indo Gulf Ferts. & Chem. Ltd.	1	—	1	20.00	69.00
6.	Rashtriya Chem. & Fert. Ltd.	5	4	9	37.9	76.98
7.	S.P.I.C.	1	—	1	15.0	66.48
8.	M.F.L.	1	—	1	25.0	20.17
9.	P.P.C.L.	1	—	1	15.0	82.00
10.	F.A.C.T.	2	1	3	38.0	71.63
11.	Zuari Agro Chem. Ltd.	2	—	2	60.0	88.52
12.	Gujarat Narmada Valley Ltd.	1	—	1	14.0	98.16
13.	Coromandal Fert. Ltd.	1	—	1	3.6	26.80
14.	Deepak Fert. Ltd.	1	—	1	9.0	69.90
15.	Chand Chap Fert. Ltd.	1	—	1	7.5	—
16.	Nagarjuna Fert. Ltd.	1	—	1	12.0	41.15
17.	KRIBHCO	—	7	7	50.0	46.93
	Total	33	32	65	603.5	54.63

The All-India Soil Testing Laboratories, its capacity number of sample analysed during the last 4 years are given in Table 8.4.

Table 8.4: Status of Soil Testing Laboratories in India during 1991-92 to 1994-95

Year	No. of Labs.			Capacity (in lakh)			% Utilisation	
	State	Industry	Total	State	Industry	Total	State	Industry
1991-92	431	87	518	59.57	7.35	66.92	76.98	64.48
1992-93	430	65	495	53.26	6.10	59.37	79.85	75.65
1993-94	432	65	497	53.45	6.10	59.55	79.19	67.39
1994-95	432	65	497	54.33	6.03	60.36	86.46	54.63

Fertiliser Recommendations

Plants take the nutrient elements (13 Nos.) from the soil, this process is called nutrient removal (Table 8.5). We have to apply fertiliser to put back the nutrients.

Because fertiliser does represent a heavy item of expenditure, the farmers in general wants to know specifically what fertiliser is best for him. He is not really interested in the "general" or "average" level of nutrients in a district or a taluka or even his village. Rather, he wants to know what kind and how much fertiliser he should use for each crop on each of his fields in each season.

Table 8.5: Plant Nutrients Removed by Some Selected Crops

Crop	Yield (kg/ha)	Nutrients removed (kg/ha)			Ratio		
		N	P_2O_5	K_2O	N	P_2O_5	K_2O
Wheat	6,000	135	65	143	100	48	106
Rice	6,000	141	60	193	100	43	137
Maize	6,000	205	87	178	100	42	87
Groundnut seed	1,906	78	22	45	100	28	58
Sugarcane	121,896	130	105	410	100	81	315
Jute	1,681	280	123	224	100	44	80
Potato	17,575	85	30	140	100	35	165

Fertiliser recommendations vary by crop, yield expected (yield goal) and soil characteristics such as nutrient test levels, soil types and basic productive capability. Recommendations may differ from state to state and from laboratory to laboratory. Ideally, fertiliser recommendations are based on research from field experiments using various rates and combinations of nutrients under all possible soil, climatic and management conditions. However, in reality, there is a limited amount of such research and this leads to different interpretations and differences of opinion and philosophies among laboratories. Thus, their fertiliser recommendations differ.

However, most of the fertiliser recommendations emanating from soil testing laboratories in India are based on soil test ratings as given in Table 8.6. Unfortunately, these rating limits are irrespective of crops and soils. Rating limits being followed in different states have been compiled in FAI.

Table 8.6: Rating Limits for Soil Test Values Traditionally Used in India

Nutrient	Low	Medium	High
Organic carbon % (as a measure of available N)	Below 0.5	0.5—0.75	above 0.75
Available N—$KMnO_4$ (kg/ha)	Below 280	280—560	above 560
Available P (kg/ha)	Below 10	10—24.6	above 24.6
Available K (kg/ha)	Below 108	108—280	above 280

The value of soil testing and its farmer acceptance can be sustained only when the fertiliser recommendations satisfy the following three types of justifications:

(a) The soil test calibration and fertiliser recommendation must be based on local field experiments which should provide significant correlation between soil test and crop response to fertilisers.

(b) The calibrations relating fertiliser recommendations to soil test values should be direct and as less subjective and qualitative as possible.

(c) The cost of soil testing should be commensurate with the precision in the estimation of fertiliser recommendation compared with cheaper alternative estimates made independent of soil testing and should increase the fertiliser use efficiency by the farmers.

It has to be recognised, therefore, that soil test research work and soil test advisory service are both like two sides of the same coin and both agencies should work in close collaboration.

Observations

While reviewing the present status of STLs in India, the following observations can be made:

(a) The number of STLs are insufficient while considering the vast cropped area.

(b) Farmers participation in the collection of soil samples are very low.

(c) Non-uniformity in the categorisation of analytical values in all the states.

(d) In most of the States, soil samples are collected only twice in a year before two main sowing seasons. Only in few States like Pondicherry, Kerala and Arunachal Pradesh, soil samples are collected throughout the year.

(e) Long period (2 months) is taken for submission of analytical reports.

(f) Recommendations mainly based on chemical characteristics of the soil and not the physical characteristics.

(g) Only few percentages of farmers follow the soil test recommendations.

9

BIOFERTILISERS IN INTEGRATED PLANT NUTRIENT SUPPLY SYSTEM A Practical Approach

— *A.K. Yadav* and *S. Raychaudhary*

INTEGRATED PLANT NUTRITION SYSTEM—A CONCEPT

Modern agriculture largely depends on the use of non-renewable fossil fuel (petroleum and coal) based inputs such as chemical fertilisers and pesticides and labour saving by using energy intensive farm machinary. Although the application of such high input technologies has undoubtedly increased production and labour efficiency but certainly on the cost of soil fertility and environment quality and has degraded some of the natural bases on which this system rests. Some of the on farm impacts of these modern technologies are:

(i) Soil erosion,
(ii) Reduction in water availability,
(iii) Salinisation and acidification of soils,
(iv) Fertiliser and pesticide contamination, and
(v) Genetic erosion.

Degradation of Soil and Environment in North-Eastern India

In the north-eastern region where although modern agricultural practices have been in use to a limited extent in plains but, not made much inroads in hilly regions. Socio-economic problems such as increase in population, requirement of land for developmental purposes and land ownership pattern, coupled with age old practices of shifting cultivation have immensely contributed to the soil and environmental degradation. Socio-economic problems, coupled with limited technology use in an imbalanced manner for immediate gains have also contributed to the problems of soil erosion and degradation, acidification of soils and genetic erosion. A huge amount of germplasm which was naturally available in this area of nature's biodiversity centre, is being lost on the pretext of introduction of new high yielding varieties.

The problem of modern resource crunch, natural resource degradation and poverty can best be illustrated by considering a rural family living in hills of north east India. Conversion of forest lands to jhuming needs of a growing population for wood, for cooking and heating have led to serious decline in the availability of fuel wood. Animal manure and crop residues may be used instead of wood, but this eliminates them from the soil as fertiliser, with concomitant reductions in crop yields and increase in erosion. Infrastructural constraints related to geographical remoteness of the area resulting into non-availability of fertilisers, poor awareness about modern agricultural practices and financial constraints do not allow them to restore the lost fertility, eventually which leads to continuous shifting of the cultivable area and cutting and degradation of forests.

Remedies and Options Available

Although the use of chemical fertilisers is the quickest and surest way of boosting crop production but due to constraints arising out of their excessive or imbalanced use in agriculturally developed areas and due to non-availability and financial constraints in underdeveloped areas

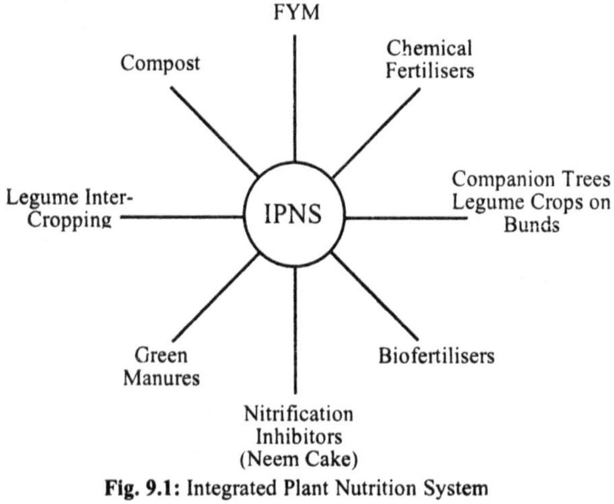

Fig. 9.1: Integrated Plant Nutrition System

(such as of North East) there seems to be no option but to fully exploit potential alternative sources of nutrients. Complimentary use of available renewable sources of plant nutrients along with chemical fertilisers in an integrated manner are of great importance not only for boosting the crop productivity but also for maintaining the soil fertility. This system is popularly known as Integrated Plant Nutrition System (IPNS).

What are Renewable Sources of Plant Nutrients

All chemical fertilisers are either mined or are based on inputs from non-renewable energy sources such as coal and petroleum. These fertilisers have known to us very recently. From centuries agriculture has flourished mainly on renewable sources of nutrients such as FYM, compost and green manuring. By definition renewable sources of nutrients mean, the nutrient sources which can be made locally in the field without the use of non-renewable inputs, using raw materials of biological origin. Renewable sources of plant nutrients are broadly classified into following categories:

RENEWABLE SOURCES OF PLANT NUTRIENTS
(ALL OF BIOLOGICAL ORIGIN)

Organic Manures	Green Manures	Legumes in cropping systems	Biofertilisers
FYM Compost Human/Animal Waste Oil cakes & Meal group of manures	Legume crop green manuring and *Azolla* green manuring	Legumes as companion crops or as intercrops	*Rhizobium* *Azotobacter* *Azospirillum* Phosphatika etc.

The Concept of IPNS vis-a-vis Other Farming Systems

To encounter the various resource and ecological constraints being faced with the introduction of chemical based, energy intensive modern agriculture, three systems are being advocated. These are:

(i) *Natural Farming System or Low External Input (LEI)*

This system envisages the use of minimum external input and stresses on better management, conservation and rotation with minimum tillage to minimise soil erosion.

(ii) *Organic Farming System*

Organic farming system is a production system which favours maximum use of organic material and discourages the use of synthetically produced agro inputs for maintaining soil fertility and productivity. Mineral grade nutrient sources such as rock phosphates are being promoted in lieu of synthetic fertilisers.

(iii) *Integrated Plant Nutrition System*

The basic concept underlying IPNS is the maintenance of soil fertility and of plant nutrient supply to an optimum level for sustaining the desired crop productivity through optimisation of benefits from all possible sources of plant nutrients.

Contrary to low external input and organic farming approach the IPNS involves a moderate external input approach complemented with available renewable resources in the form of organic manures, green manures and biofertilisers to obtain a targetted yield, based not only on cropping and farming system, but also on distinct geographical areas or villages as a dynamic system. The best associations of various types of plant nutrients in different fields are identified for a balanced plant nutrition and high yield. For renewable sources of organic origin either locally available material of plant and animal origin (*e.g.*, washings) be used or *in situ* production of organics be attempted. In hills, where non-cultivated areas are abundantly available, biomass production be attempted for transfer of nutrients to cultivated areas. In plains and valleys where land is scarce, biomass production in fallows and on borders be attempted.

Among other alternative potential sources, are quick growing leguminous shrubs, trees and forage and food legumes. To strengthen the potential of legumes, they be invariably inoculated with *Rhizobium* inoculants.

Among biofertilisers, use of *Rhizobium* in legumes, *Azotobacter* and *Azospirillum* in non-legumes, Blue green algae and *Azolla* in rice and phosphatika in all crops have been found to be highly effective. Due importance should be given to inoculants in compost making for obtaining enriched compost.

A Model Example of IPNS in Plains in Rice Crop

Total nutrient requirement 80 : 40 : 40 :: NPK.

1. Grow food legume such as french bean or cowpea duly inoculated with *Rhizobium* inoculant during summer after first showers.
2. Harvest the first flush of pods and utilise as green vegetables.
3. Incorporate the entire legume crop into soil after cutting and ploughing.
4. Use only 40 kg N, 30 kg P_2O_5 and 30 kg K_2O as chemical fertiliser.
5. Treat paddy seedling roots with *Azospirillum* inoculants.
6. Transplant paddy seedlings.
7. After 7-8 days of planting add fresh *Azolla* @ 500 kg/ha to standing crop.
8. The resultant yield will be higher than the 100 per cent NPK control.

A model example of IPNS in Hills in Vegetable Crop

1. Prepare enriched compost using forest litter/paddy straw and animal wastes, microbial inoculants and rock phosphate.
2. Incorporate compost @ 8-10 tons/ha in the field.
3. Treat vegetable seedlings with *Azotobacter* inoculant as seedling root dip or soil treatment in case of potato or ginger.
4. Use 50 per cent N, 60 per cent P_2O_5 and 50 per cent K_2O of recommended doses as chemical fertiliser.
5. The resultant yield will be comparable to 100 per cent NPK control.

BIOLOGICAL SYSTEMS OF NUTRIENT MOBILISATION

The major nutrients required in crop cultivation are nitrogen, phosphorus and potash. Besides these three, there are several other nutrients which are required in minor to micro quantities. N, P and K are provided to the soil, which is the basic medium of cultivation, through three different processes. These are:

(a) By chemical fertilisers.
(b) By organic manures.
(c) By biological mobilising systems either already present in the soil or added artificially in the form of biofertilisers.

Other minor and micro nutrients are being supplied mainly either from the decomposition of the organic matter or from soil's natural reserve.

Biological nutrient mobilisation has attracted lot of attention during the last four decades and attempts were made to exploit these systems to harness their best benefits. As a result of massive research, three systems have been identified for large scale adoption. These are:

(a) Biological Nitrogen Fixation system.
(b) Phosphate solubilisation/mobilisation system.
(c) Compost acceleration and enrichment system.

A. Biological Nitrogen Fixation

Biological fixation of elemental atmospheric nitrogen is a unique property of some prokaryots, *viz.* Bacteria and Cyanobacteria. These organisms (known as diazotrophs) possess a unique enzyme complex known as Nitrogenase, which is responsible for this character. Included in the list are free living species of *Azotobacter, Azospirillum, Kiebsiella*, photosynthetic bacteria, cyanobacteria and bacteria that can fix N_2 only under symbiotic associationship such as *Rhizobium*. Few other symbiotic associationships are of *Azolla-Anabaena* and *Franida*—some tree species. nodulation by *Rhizobium* in legumes is the most important source of biologically fixed nitrogen in agriculture and it offers the greatest potential for genetic improvement in the long-term. A list of important N_2 fixing micro-organism is given in diagram.

Nitrogen Fixation in the Biosphere

The atmospheric nitrogen which constitutes the basic N reservoir for all biological and industrial system occupies the major portion of the atmospheric air (75% by weight and 78% by volume) and is being fixed or converted into usable form by three methods:

(a) By Natural electrical lightening and precipitation,
(b) By industrial N_2 fixation, and
(c) Through biological nitrogen fixation.

About the total quantum of nitrogen being fixed in the entire earth, there are divergent views among scientists. Keeping in view of the most widely accepted opinion it has been estimated that approximately 180-200 million tons of N_2 is being fixed on the entire earth per year, out of which, natural lightning and precipitation account for merely 5 per cent (10 million tons), industrial nitrogen fixation contribute 20 per cent (40 million tons) and biological nitrogen fixation accounts for remaining 75 per cent (175 million tons).

IMPORTANT N_2 FIXING MICRO-ORGANISMS

Free living diazotrophs	Symbiotic diazotroph	Associative diazotrophs
(a) *Strict anaerobes* Clostridium Desulfo-vibrio	(a) *Rhizobium-Legume* Rhizobium Bradytrizobium Azotrizobium	Azotobacter with Graminae plants Azospirillum with Graminae plants Acetobacter with sugarcane plants
(b) *Facultative anaerobes* Kiebsiella Enterobacter	(b) *Franida-Non-legumes*	
(c) *Micro aerobes* Aquasprillum Arthrobacter Azosprillum	(c) *Anabaena Azollae-Azolla*	
(d) *Arobes* Azotobacter Beijerinckia derxia		
(e) *Photosynthetic* Rhodosprillum Chromatium		
(f) *Cyanobacteria* Anabaena Nostoc Scytonema		

In biological nitrogen fixation, the contribution of different systems are given in Table 9.1.

Harvesting Biological Nitrogen Fixation for Agriculture

As per Subba Rao (1979 and 1993) there are two, conventional and novel approaches to this problem. Under conventional approach initially the strategies involving legume—*Rhizobium* systems were incorporated, but later during last two decades few more strategies involving other N_2 fixing systems have also been added. These are:

Table 9.1: Biological Nitrogen Fixation, the Contribution of Different Systems

Sources	Quantity (million tons)
Legume crops	35
Non-legumes	9
Permanent grassland	45
Forest & Woodland	40
Unused land	10
Sea	36
Total	175

Source: Burris (1997) and Burns & Hardy (1975).

Conventional Approach

1. Increase area under cultivation of legumes.
2. Provide efficient strains of Rhizobia for inoculating legumes.
3. Provide efficient strains of other non-symbiotic nitrogen fixers for inoculating cereals, millets, vegetables and cash crops.
4. Evolve highly competitive strains of N_2 fixing organisms, so that they can compete with inefficient native population.
5. Evolve appropriate strains and application methodologies for use in problematic soils such as acidic soils of N.E. Region.
6. Overcome inhibition of chemical N on biological nitrogen fixation.
7. Encourage the use of green manuring practices in different cropping systems.
8. Define agronomic practices leading to conservation of moisture and nitrogen for better nodulation and nitrogen fixation.

Novel Approach

1. Induce nodulation in cereals and other non-legumes.
2. Increase the range of nitrogen fixing organisms in the soil by implanting "nif" gene from N_2 fixing bacteria to non-nitrogen fixing bacteria.
3. Implant nitrogen fixation capacity from N_2 fixing bacteria tc crop plants by protoplast fusion and tissue culture.
4. Find out new N_2 fixing associations among plants and harness them to agriculture.
5. Synthesize nitrogenase enzyme and use in N_2 fixation as a catalyst in industrial processes.

Mechanism of B.N.F.

The nitrogenase enzyme complex, which is found in all N_2 fixing micro-organisms is the most important component of BNF process. The enzyme complex is made up of two components one with iron and molybdenum having a molecular weight of 200,000 and the second with only iron having a molecular weight of 65,000. Other requirements of the process are:

(a) Anaerobic environment around nitrogenase.
(b) Hydrogen ions as $NaDH_2$ or $NaDPH_2$.
(c) Nitrogen gas.
(d) Energy in the form of ATP.
(e) Reduced electron through electron carriers.

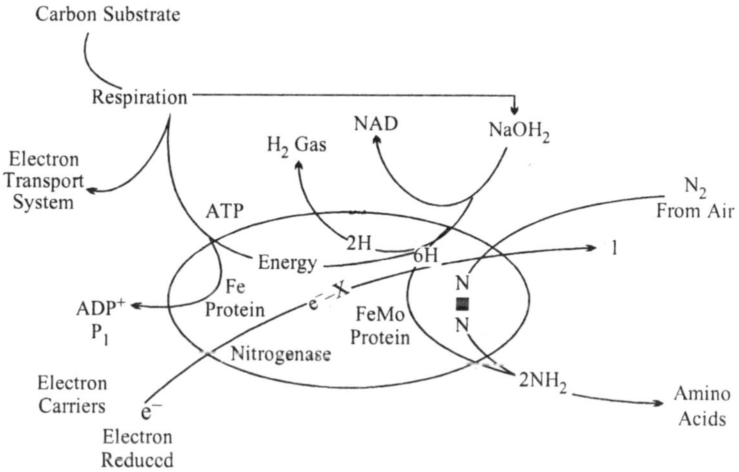

Fig. 9.2: Mechanism of N_2 Fixation

Sources of all these requirements may differ in different BNF systems. But the site of N_2 fixation is always the bacterial cell. The schematic representation of the mechanism of N_2 fixation is given in Fig. 9.2.

B. Phosphate Solubilisation

After nitrogen, phosphorus is second most sought after nutrient. Although most of the Indian soils do have poor to moderate phosphorus as soil reserve, but this is practically of no use to plants, as it is present in fixed or insoluble forms. From P availability point of view most of the Indian soils are deficient to highly deficient in available P. The situation is much more serious in the N.E. Region, where most of the soils which are acidic to highly acidic in nature, not only keep the soil's reserve phosphorus into fixed form but also render applied phosphorus into insoluble form within a short period of time. All phosphorus ions either as primary orthophosphate ions or as secondary phosphate ions are subjected to fixation with hydroxides of Aluminium and Iron. In hills, where soils are rich in organic matter, the P availability is comparatively better. It is mainly due to microbial activity. These organisms secrete various types of acidic metabolites, which bring about change in soil pH and release P from organic and inorganic complexes. At higher altitudes the scenario is again grim due to prevailing low temperature and low microbial activity.

Studies made in soils with poor to rich in organic carbon, have invariably revealed that the microbial activity leading to release of P may be low to moderate in soils, depending upon the organic carbon contents, but the activity in rhizosphere of growing plants keep on going without much difference. This activity of root associated bacteria, fungi and to some extent mycorrhizal fungi, which extend plant rhizosphere, help in solubilisation and absorption of phosphorus. The theme of using these bacteria and fungi as phosphate solubilising systems have originated from this knowledge.

A large number of heterotrophic and autotrophic soil micro-organisms are known to have the capacity to solubilise inorganic phosphates through their metabolic activity. A list of such important phosphate solubilising micro-organisms are given in diagram.

IMPORTANT PHOSPHATE SOLUBILISING MICRO-ORGANISMS

- Phosphate solubilisers
  - Bacteria
    - *Bacillus* sp.
    - *Pseudomonas* sps.
    - *Flavobacterium* sps.
    - *Xanthomonas* sps
    - *Nitrosomonas*
    - *Nitrobacter*
    - *Thiobacillus* sps.
  - Fungi
    - *Aspergillus* species
    - *Penicillium*
    - *Curvularia lunata*
    - *Fusarium oxysporium*
    - *Cladosporium*
    - *Rhizoctonia*
  - Actinomycetes
    - *Actinomyces*
    - *Streptomyces*
- Phosphate absorbers
  - V.A. Mycorrhiza
    - *Glomus*
    - *Gigaspora*
    - *Enterophospora*
    - *Scierocystis*
    - *Scutellospora*

Intensive studies made by different groups of scientists during the last three decades have identified some selected species and strains of bacteria, fungi and mycorrhizal fungi which are not only capable of solubilising the fixed phosphorus in the soil but are also quite competent to multiply rapidly in rhizospheric region of targetted plants, even in soils poor in organic carbon. Various combinations of bacteria and fungi have been suggested to suit the different soil conditions in different region.

Mechanism of Phosphate Solubilisation

Production of carbon dioxide, hydrogen sulphide, mineral acids and organic acids by selected group of micro-organisms are the major factors responsible for solubilisation of fixed phosphorus in the soil. Out of these, production of organic acid is the most important factor compared to other ones.

All the micro-organisms which play significant role in P solubilisation are free living and grow rapidly in the presence of organic matter, irrespective of the type of plants and crops. They are also capable of growing vigorously in rhizospheric region of growing roots. Herein their normal course of metabolic activities, they secrete various extra-cellular metabolites such as CO_2, H_2S, H_2SO_4, HNO_3 and organic acids etc., which are responsible in P solubilisation. Higher the population of such micro-organisms in the rhizospheric region, higher will be the P solubilisation in an area near the roots, from where these soluble P ions can be absorbed by plants.

Various reactions involved in phosphate solubilisation through microbial activities are as follows:

(a) CO_2 solubilisation:

$$Ca_3(PO_4)_2 + CO_2 + H_2O \longrightarrow 2CaHPO_4 + CaCO_3$$

$$Ca_3(PO_4)_2 + 2CO_2 + 2H_2O \longrightarrow Ca(H_2PO_4)_2 + 2CaCO_3$$

(b) Mineral acid solubilisation:

$$Ca_3(PO_4)_2 + 2HNO_3 \xrightarrow[\text{Bacteria}]{\text{Nitrifying}} 2CaHPO_4 + Ca(NO_3)_2$$

$$Ca_3(PO_4)_2 + H_2SO_4 \xrightarrow[\text{Such as } \textit{Thiobacillus}]{\text{Sulphur bacteria}} CaHPO_4 + CaSO_4$$

(c) H_2S solubilisation:

$$FePO_4 + H_2S \xrightarrow[\text{as } \textit{Desulfo-vibrio}]{\text{Bacteria such}} FeS + H_2PO_4^-$$

(d) Organic acid solubilisation:

$Ca_3(PO_4)_2$ or $FePO_4$ or $AlPO_4$

Organic acids such as citric acid, oxalic, lactic, malic, tarteric & α-ketogluteric

CHELATION

Stable organic Complexes of Ca^{++}, Fe^{+++} & Al^{+++}

H_2PO_4 primary & secondary orthophosphate ions

C. Compost Acceleration and Enrichment

Production of organic manures such as FYM and compost is basically a microbiological process accomplished by the combined activity of bacteria, fungi, Actinomycetes and protozoa which are present in the composting material. The quality and nutrient value of the final product, very much depend upon the material composted, addition of additives and combination of micro-organisms. A list of important micro-organisms being used as compost accelerators and enrichers are given in Table 9.2.

Table 9.2: List of Compost Accelerating and Enriching Micro-Organisms

Compost Accelerators			
(i)	Cellulolytic fungi	:	*Aspergillus, Chaetomium, Penicillium Fusarium, Trichoderma, Paecilliomyces*
	Cellulolytic bacteria	:	*Bacillus, Cellulomonas, Clostridium, Cytophaga, Pseudomonas*
(ii)	Lignolytic fungi	:	*Clavaria, Cephalosporium, Humicol*
	Lignolytic bacteria	:	*Pseudomonas, Flavobacterium*
Compost Enrichers			
	N_2-Fixer	:	*Azotobacter, Clostridium*
	P-Solubiliser	:	*Cellulomonas, Asperigillus, Penicillium*

To enrich the compost and to reduce the composting time various additives and microbial inoculants have been developed which on using in compost pits along with composting materials not only reduce the time by 2 to 4 weeks but also increase its nutrient value to a significantly higher level. Paddy straw compost prepared by traditional composting methods contains 0.5 to 0.9 per cent N, 0.1 to 0.2 per cent P_2O_5 and 0.3 to 0.5 per cent K_2O with a C/N ratio of 24 : 1. Enriched compost prepared from same paddy straw using compost accelerating inoculants, P solubilising inoculants, N_2 fixing inoculants and Rock phosphate, provide 1.8 per cent N, 0.3 per cent P_2O_5 and 0.5 per cent K_2O with a C/N ratio of 16 : 1.

BIOFERTILISERS

The term biofertiliser is made up of two words. "Bio" means living, and "fertiliser" means a product which provide nutrients in usable form. Put together Biofertiliser means a living product which provide nutrients to the crop. But as a product biofertiliser does not contain any significant quantity of nutrients in itself, it contains mainly live bacterial or fungal cells, which on application, help in fixing or solubilising the nutrients present in air or in soil.

As discussed in earlier chapters that in nature there are some micro-organisms present in the soil which help in fixation of N_2, solubilisation of phosphorus and degradation of complex organic matter. The quantum of nutrient mobilisation by these organisms very much depends upon their population in the soil or in rhizospheric region of the roots. Under normal circumstances the soil possesses a complex mixture of wide range of micro-organisms, out of them only a few help in nutrient mobilisation. If proper benefits of this biological system is to be harvested, then it is essential to increase the population of such specified micro-organisms by artificial inoculation. Biofertilisers are ready to use live formulations of such micro-organisms. Biofertilisation technology basically involves three steps. These are:

(1) Identification and selection of such beneficial micro-organisms.
(2) Mass multiplication of such micro-organisms in laboratories and industries to prepare usable formulations.
(3) Artificial inoculation of these microbial formulations in soil through seeds or seedlings to increase their population to an acceptable threshold limit for a significant period of time.

Strictly going by definition the biofertilisers are ready to use, live formulations of some specific and effective strains of micro-organisms, which on application to seed, seedling root or soil help in mobilisation of nutrients from their natural, non-available forms to available forms (which plants can absorb directly) through their biological activity. For example *Azotobacter, Azospirillum.* Blue green algae etc. fix atmospheric nitrogen and enrich the soil. *Rhizobium* in association with legume fix atmospheric N and provide to their host. Organisms like *Bacillus, Pseudomonas, Aspergillus* etc. secrete organic acids which solubilise fixed phosphorus present in the soil and convert it into primary and secondary orthophosphate ions. Similarly some other micro-organisms such as *Trichoderma, Chaetomium, Myrothecium* etc. act on complex organic matter and release a wide range of nutrients from their captivity.

Different Types of Biofertilisers

Biofertilisers or microbial inoculants as manageable agricultural inputs were introduced in India as early as 1934. But till early seventies they received very little attention and it was only *Rhizobium* which was being produced in a few laboratories. With the introduction of Soybean cultivation during 1968 to 1975 people realised the importance of *Rhizobium* biofertiliser and to fulfil the demand, lot of production units were established during late seventies to early eighties. Initially the entire attention was on *Rhizobium* but since late eighties, new and new biofertilisers were added to the list of greatly diversified subject. Since then consistently new microbial systems are being added. Depending upon their activity of mobilising different nutrients, biofertilisers are being classified as in the diagram.

POTENTIAL OF DIFFERENT BIOFERTILISERS

Table 9.3: Potential of N_2 Fixing Microbial Inoculants

Sl.No.	Biofertiliser and Associated Crops	Potential of B, N, P in kg/ha	Potantiality of Fertiliser N Replacement kg/ha	% Increase due to Inoculation over Control
1.	*Rhizobium* in symbiosis with legumes	50-300	20-40	10-60
2.	*Azotobacter* in rhizosphere of non-legume upland crops	25-40	15-25	10-25
3.	*Azospirillum* as associative symbiont with non-legumes	25-40	15-30	20-35
4.	Blue green algae in low land rice fields	25-40	20-30	10-20
5.	*Acetobacter* as associative symbiont with sugarcane	30-150	60-100	25-50

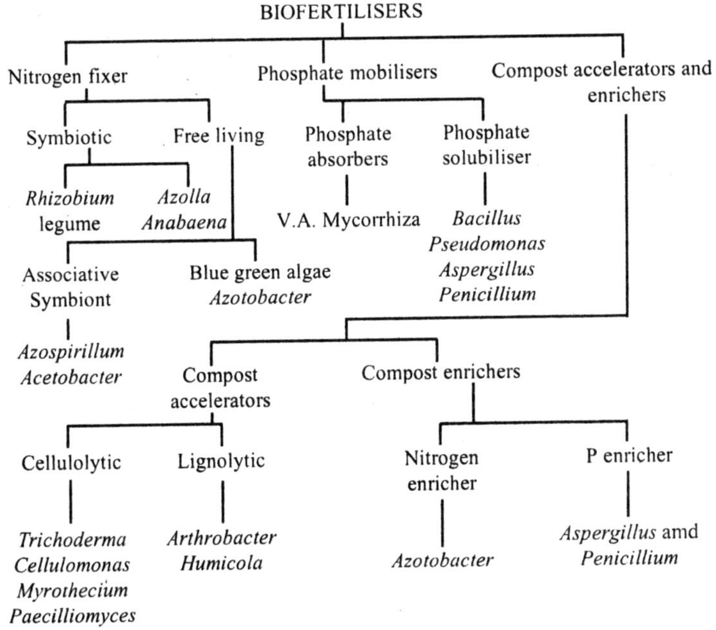

Table 9.4: Potential of Rhizobium Inoculated Green Manuring Crop on Incorporation in the Field

Sl.No.	Green Manuring Crop	Output in 45-80 days	
		Green matter Incorporated ton/ha	N Contribution in kg/ha
1.	Sunhemp (*Crotolaria juncea*)	21.2	91
2.	*Sesbania acculeata*	20.2	86
3.	*Vigna sinensis* (cowpea)	15.0	74
4.	*Sesbania rostrata*	24.0	120

Table 9.5: Potential of Azolla Green Manuring in Low Land Rice

Sl.No.	Manuring in low land	Green matter Incorporated ton/ha	N enrich of soil in kg/ha	Fertiliser N replacement in kg/ha
1.	Azolla as basal green manure	10-12	50-60	30-35
2.	As dual cropping single dose inoculation @ 500 kg/ha	5-6	25-30	15-20
3.	As dual cropping two doses @ 500 kg/ha	8-10	40-50	20-30
4.	Both as basal green manure and dual cropping	16-20	80-100	60-65

Table 9.6: Potential of Phosphate solubilising inoculant (Phosphatika) (Potentiality of P Solubilisation in Laboratory in mg/15 gm Insoluble P/15 gm Sucrose)

Sl.No.	Inoculant	P Solubilisation Potential in mg
1.	*Pseudomonas striata*	78
2.	*Bacillus polymyxa*	83
3.	*Aspergillus awamorii*	138
4.	*Penicillium digitatum*	152
5.	Mixture of all above	166

Potential of phosphatika inoculant on crop yield and P_2O_5 uptake have been found to be increasing the efficiency of applied phosphorus by 15-20 per cent. It phosphatika inoculants were used with 50 per cent of recommended dose of P_2O_5 as SSP and 50 per cent Rock phosphate, yield remain at par with crop applied with 100 per cent P_2O_5 as single superphosphate (SSP).

Phosphatika inoculant on application with other N_2 fixing biofertilisers have been found to be not only improving the P availability but were also encouraging the N_2 fixing capability of N_2 fixers.

Potential of Compost Accelerators and Enrichers

Application of compost accelerator inoculants such as *Trichoderma viridi* and *Paecilliomyces fusisporus*, tremendously improve the C/N ratio from 33 : 1 of control to 22 : 1. Application of compost enrichers such as phosphate solubilising inoculants (*Aspergillus awamorii*) along with rock phosphate and N_2 fixing inoculants (Azotobacter) have been found to be reducing the C/N ratio further down to 16 : 1. Total available phosphorus was found to be increased from 0.15 per cent in control to 0.3 per cent in compost provided with compost accelerators and enrichers both.

Total time period required for composting was also found to be reduced by 2-4 weeks.

Advantages of Using Biofertilisers

* Can replace 20 to 50 per cent of chemical fertiliser N and 15-25 per cent of synthetic phosphatic fertilisers.
* Biofertilisers being cheap, provide highly cost effective supplement of chemical fertilisers.
* Increase farm productivity. Generally 10-40 per cent in grain yield and 15-30 per cent in vegetative growth.

* Activates soil biologically thereby increasing natural fertility of soil.
* Help in stimulating plant growth in general and roots in particular as they secrete various growth promoting substances, hormones and vitamins. They help in better nutrient uptake and increased tolerance towards drought and moisture stress.
* Some biofertiliser organisms also secrete some fungistatic and antibiotic like substances, which reduce the incidence of certain diseases and increases disease resistance.
* Help in decomposing plant residues in soil, thereby improving C/N ratio in soil, improving soil texture and structure. Also help in increasing water holding capacity.
* In composting processes improve the quality and nutrient value of the compost.
* Being environment friendly and cost effective do not cause any harmful effect on soil and environment. On the contrary they help in degradation of other harmful chemicals such as weedicides and pesticides. Thereby they help in increasing the biodegradation capability of the soil.

REFERENCES

Burns, R.C. and Hardy, R.W.F. (1975). *Nitrogen Fixation in Bacteria and High Plants*, Springer Verlag, New York.

Burris, R.H. (1977). *Overview of Nitrogen Fixation In Genetic Engineering for Nitrogen Fixation* (Ed. Hallaender, A.), Plenum Press, New York, pp. 8-18.

Subba Rao, N.S. (1977). *Soil Micro-Organisms and Plant Growth*, Oxford & IBH Publishing Co., New Delhi.

Subba Roa, N.S. (1993). *Biofertiliser in Agriculture and Forestry*, Oxford & IBH Publishing Co., New Delhi.

10

DEVELOPMENT AND USE OF BIOFERTILISERS IN PRESENT DAY FERTILISER SCENARIO

— *A.K. Yadav*

The population on earth is expected to reach around 6253 million by 2000 A.D. About 2600 million tons of cereals and 520 million tons of grain legumes will be needed to constitute just part of the food required to feed this increased growth of population. Prospects of meeting nitrogen requirements in India through the creation of new fertiliser plants are not good because of the cost of machinery, the rising cost of natural gas or Naptha and the lack of less energy consuming industrial processes other than the Haber-Bosch process to convert nitrogen and hydrogen into ammonia. In countries with advanced technologies energy requirements for heating, living and working premises, mechanised agriculture and the maintenance of industrial production lines are so great that alternative methods for augmenting soil fertility to raise grain crops will soon become necessary. At present, the pinch on fertiliser consumption is felt more by the developing nations which cannot afford to import plant nutrients at high price.

Moreover Nitrogen is a unique element in that, there is almost no nitrogen present in mineral form in nature and yet above every hectare of soil at sea level, there are 78 million kg. of inert nitrogen gas. Plants, as eucaryotic autotroph need an oxidized or reduced form of Nitrogen for anabolism. The energy cost of biological nitrogen fixation is significant. Currently 1-2 per cent of the world's fossil energy is used for fertiliser while about 1-2 billion ton of plant carbohydrate from photosynthesis is consumed in biological nitrogen fixation.

The ability of procaryotic organisms to reduce atmospheric nitrogen to usable forms has been known for over 100 years. It is generally estimated that biological nitrogen fixation accounts for about 175 MT of fixed nitrogen per year compared with about 80 MT of ammonia produced annually through the Haber process. 75 per cent of which is available for fertiliser. Thus the most important yield of fixed nitrogen result from biological nitrogen fixation. So the need for exploiting these biological agents is felt very much at this present juncture.

There are mainly two types of Biological Nitrogen Fixation occurs in nature.

Symbiosis and Asymbiosis

The term symbiosis generally denotes a mutual beneficial partnership between organisms.

Main symbiotic Nitrogen fixer is *Rhizobium* which is used extensively throughout the world for leguminous crops, *viz*. pulses and oilseeds (groundnut and soybean).

Here Symbiosis occurs between the *Rhizobium* and the leguminous plant. Rhizobia enter the roots of legumes either through root hair or directly. The manifestation of infection is the appearance in root hairs of an infection thread and the bacteria goes interior of the root where it forms nodule. The nodule is merely a protective tissue where the bacteria live in and supply ammonia to the host plant.

The effectiveness of the nodulation could be easily distinguished by the colour of the nodule, if the colour is pink then the nodule is efficient one and fix nitrogen directly from air. It should always be kept in mind that the *Rhizobium* are very much host specific. One specics of *Rhizobium* can form nodule to a specific leguminous group and do not in others.

Azotobacter, Azospirillum and Blue Green Algae

Azotobacter is a free living non-symbiotic nitrogen fixer and *Azospirillum* is an associative symbiont since they occur in cortical cells and phytoxylem vessels as endosysbionts.

In low land rice field BGA (Blue Green Algae) has a major contribution in nitrogen economy of the soil. Besides the above nitrogen fixing free living organisms there are some more agriculturally important micro-organism like phosphorous solubulising bacteria and cellulose and lignin decomposers which are also used as biofertiliser for their specific role.

Phosphobactrin

As most of the inorganic applied phosphorus are chemically fixed within 48 hrs in the soil, the need of phosphobactria have been felt very much in recent years. The insoluble chemically fixed phosphorus is being slowly released by these bacteria which help the standing crop to spread its root zone and subsequent uptake of nutrient resulting in increase of yield.

Cellulose and Lignin Decomposers

Continuous application of inorganic fertiliser in the long run destroy the soil physical structure as well as increase the pollution in the environment. So the use of organic manure is very much needed in this present situation. Conversion of farm waste, city waste and other domestic refuse to organic manures with the help of cellulose and lignin decomposers help the environment by keeping it not only pollution free as well as restore the physical and chemical health of soils and increase the yield to a greater extent.

Production

Specific effective strains of micro organisms are collected from reputed research institutes or universities and multiply in the specific medium up to a cell concentration of 10^9—10^{10}/ml. This rich harvested cell broth is then mixed with a sterilised carrier material to obtain a final cell count of 10^8 cell/gm. The poly packed biofertiliser is then kept at 20-28°C for 2 days and then sent to the dealers point. The polypacked material should be marked with the expiry date as the organisms itself has a shelf life period upto 4 to 6 months. The users are advised not to use the biofertiliser after expiry date.

Agronomic Result

The nitrogen fixing biofertilisers are now used extensively in the farmers field and it has been shown that 20-30 per cent increase of the yield over control. Many field researcher have been conducted in different fields throughout the country. The result of some are given in the Table 10.1.

Besides nitrogen contribution in the standing crop *Rhizobium, Azotobacter* and *Azospirillum* excrete plant auxns mainly IAA (Indole Acetic Acid) for root and stem elongatiom. Moreover, they also excrete

Table 10.1: Response of Biofertiliser on Some Important Crops in North East Region

Sl.No.	Crops	Biofertiliser Used	Total No of Trials Conducted	Range of Increase in Yield Due to Biofertiliser over Control	Average Increase in Yield Due to Biofertiliser
1.	Paddy	*Azospirillum* & PSM	30 Nos.	5.50 — 43.50	16.80
2.	Maize	*Azospirillum* & PSM	5 Nos.	8.10 — 15.10	12.58
3.	Wheat	*Azotobacter* & PSM	5 Nos.	4.10 — 17.40	10.33
4.	Mustard	*Azotobacter* & PSM	14 Nos.	4.04 — 26.66	11.77
5.	Potato	*Azotobacter* & PSM	6 Nos.	7.21 — 17.14	10.08
6.	Pea	*Rhizobium* & PSM	26 Nos.	8.81 — 26.19	22.87
7.	Lentil	*Rhizobium* & PSM	17 Nos.	12.50 — 37.55	22.45
8.	Fr. Bean (Green Pods)	*Rhizobium* & PSM	7 Nos.	8.46 — 21.70	12.13
9.	Fr. Bean (Grains)	*Rhizobium* & PSM	2 Nos.	11.11 — 25.00	18.05
10.	Ground Nut	*Rhizobium* & PSM	4 Nos.	10.50 — 27.50	16.78

some antifungal and antibacterial toxin during their metabolic pathway. So from the disease control point of view the biofertiliser has great role in crop management.

It has also been observed that in winter legume *Azospirillum* along with *Rhizobium* respond significantly than *Rhizobium* alone.

Dose

Unlike chemical fertilisers or pesticides biofertiliser has no fixed dose as more population more the chance of survival in the Rhizosphere. Generally, it is recommended that 4.5 g. of Biofertiliser is enough to treat one kg of seeds. But the dose may vary according to field situation like moisture content, soil temperature, etc.

Constraint

Mainly soil pH, soil temperature, soil moisture, etc. are the major constraints for applied biofertiliser.

Conclusion

Owing to the intensive farming and introduction of HYV mainly in cereals the use of inorganic fertiliser increased very much. As a result the physical structure, underground water as well as environment have been tremendously deteriorated day by day. Again misuse and overuse of fertiliser is a serious concern to the national economy.

In this grave situation biofertiliser shows us some light of hope. It though not fully but supplement the part of the nitrogen requirement of the HYV crop and maintain soil physical structure, pollution free environment and soil ecology. On the other hand the resource poor farmer could get the benefit of the biofertiliser at a minimum investment and reap the harvest at a substantial amount to feed his family.

11

NEEM AS AN INTEGRATED SOURCE OF NUTRIENTS IN THE MANAGEMENT OF CROP PRODUCTION

— *R.C. Gupta, N.P. Singh* and *D.N. Upadhyay*

Abstract

With a increase in population pressure, various multiple cropping systems have become popular in different parts of country. Similarly, from the use of single nutrient, application of multiple nutrient become a rule. No single sources of plant nutrient (organic, biological or chemical) can satisfy the need of all the essential elements that the crop needs for its growth and development. Therefore, superimposition of all the sources of plant nutrients on different cropping systems is being attempted to provide balanced nutrients to increase crop productivity and plant nutrient use efficiency. Neem stands on this.

Neem tree has remained a integral part of human eco-systems in India. Increasing environmental pollution and hazardous effects caused to air, soil and water and to the whole living world by inorganic fertilisers and pesticides have created global concern among the future thinkers of the world. It has now already drawn the attention of Scientists for search of biofertilisers and biopesticides. In this search, Neem (*Azadirachta indica*) has been identified as a wonder plant because of its multispecturm usefulness in almost every aspect of human activity. However, the present paper elucidate potentialities of Neem as biofertilisers and improving Nitrogen efficiency.

Introduction

Neem tree occurs predominantly in dry deciduous regions in its natural habitat. It is planted on roadsides, village homesteads, bunds and farm boundaries for its multifarious uses. For nearly the past two decades, neem has come under close scientific scrutiny as a source of novel, natural biopesticide and biofertiliser.

Neem is native to Burma and the arid regions of the Indian sub-continent, where it is almost been semi-domesticated. During the last century, neem has also been introduced in arid zones of Africa. Today, it is grown in many Asian countries, in tropical regions of New World, in several Caribbean and in some Mediterranean countries. During the last decades, neem has been introduced and planted on a large scale in Philippines and in plains of Arafat near Meccah in Saudi Arabia, in regions ecologically highly diverse. In all these areas, the tree is thriving a testimony to its hardiness and adaptability. Neem, however, is unsuited to growing in cooler and mountainous areas (> 1000 m). There are an estimated 14 million neem trees distributed in different parts of the India. Though the plant is adapted to a wide range of climates, it thrives well in tropical and subtropical conditions. The tree grows in almost all types of soils, but it prefers well drained alkaline soils. Neem has not been found to grow well in north-eastern region of India except in Lumding area of Assam. However, Maha-neem (*Melia azedarach*) was found growing very well throughout the north east region (NE region).

Since ancient times, neem has been associated with healing in the subcontinent of India. Its botanical name, *Azadirachta indica*, derived from Farsi, azad darakhat in Hindi literally means "the tree of the Indian subcontinent." Neem's Sanskritized name "Arishta" means reliever of sickness. In Kiswaili, neem is known as "Mwarubaini" reliever of 40 disorders. The early Ayurvedic literature, especially "Charak Samhita" and the Unani system of medicine, document neem's medicinal and therapeutic uses. Even in Africa, tropical America, and the other parts of the world, where neem has been introduced in recent times, people have learnt of neem as herbal treatments for various ailments. A large number of medicinal, cosmetics, toiletries and pharmaceutical are now based on neem products.

Neem remained one of the versatile and multipurpose tree. Neem tree with its pleasant shade and cooling effect had always attracted the Indian people. People take rest during hot sun under the neem tree.

It is much loved by Indian God and Goddess specially the seven sisters, Goddess Kali and Shitala Devi. Neem in Indian culture has been ranked higher than "Kalpa Vriksha," the mythological, wish fulfilling tree. In "Sharh-e-Mufridat,"Al-Qanoon, Neem has been named as "Shafar-e-Mukarak," "the blessed tree" because of its highly beneficial properties. Though scientific studies are needed, neem is reported to purify air and the environment of noxious elements. Its shade not only cools but prevents many diseases. During hot summer months in northern parts of the subcontinent the temperature under the neem is –10°C less than the surrounding temperature; 10 air-conditioners operated together may not do the job as efficiently and economically as a full grown neem.

About a decade ago, some 50,000 neem trees were planted over 10 km^2 on the plains of Arafat to provide shade for Muslim pilgrims during Haj. It is an ancient belief that neem growing inside the house can keep the surrounding air clean of impurities and thereby control environmental pollution. Also, hanging neem twigs on the door of a house is said to offer protection against pollution.

The interest in neem tree in the developed world is attributed to the fact that neem-based pest control products in the diverse modes of action are not only effective against pests, but also inherently defer, less persistent in environment, and less prone to the problem of pest resistance than the synthetics. The tree is not only beautiful to look at, but full grown neem trees yield between 10 to 100 tonnes of dried bio-mass ha^{-1}, depending on rainfall, site characteristics, spacing, ecotype or genotype; fruits and woods constitute one quarter each. Improved management of neem stands can yield harvests of about 12.5 cubic metre (40 tonnes) of high quality solid wood ha^{-1}. This evergreen perennial tree can survive up from 200 to 300 years, if not cut down. India has an estimated 14 million neem trees producing about 8 lakh tonnes of seed annually. Nearly 100 oil mills and 40 biopesticide units consume more than 8 lakh tonnes of seed annually.

In present time scientists, all over the world, are very much concerned for increasing pollution in air, soil and water. The extensive and intensive use of inorganic fertilisers for maximum agricultural crop production indirectly leaves residual toxic substances in food which is taken by animals as well as human beings. The chemicals used as fertilisers, constitute specially the micro-nutrients, viz. nitrogen, phosphorus and potash providing nutrients for growth and health of the plants and utilised as urea, ammonium sulphate, ammonium phosphate, muriate of potash, potassium sulphate and super phosphate etc.

The increasing pesticides and inorganic chemicals toxicity in our body has alarmed and cautioned us to think, which resulted in the form of as sustainable agriculture and it calls for use of eco-friendly biofertilisers and biopesticides. Among several plants products which have been investigated for their utilisation as fertilisers Neem tree is one of them. In view of the vision for sustainable development and sustainable agriculture, the importance of Neem with its potentialities as biofertiliser is increasing day by day.

Physical Nature of Neem

Neem is an evergreen, tall fast growing tree which can reach a height of

25 m and 2.5 m in girth. It has an attractive crown of deep-green foliage (which can spread 10 m. across) and mosses of honey-scented flowers. The tree thrives even on nutrient-poor dry soil. It tolerated high to very high temperatures, low rainfall, long spells of drought, and salinity. It is propagated by seed, 9 to 12 months old seedlings transplant well. Birds and fruits bats also disperse the seed. Fruiting begins, in 3 to 5 years. In the Indian subcontinent, neem flowers from January through April, some off-types also fruits in November or December, the fruit is about 2 cm long and, when ripe, has a yellow fleshy pericarp, a white hard shell, and a brown, oil-rich seed kernal. Fruits yields ranges from 30 to 100 kg per tree depending on rainfall insolation, soil type, and neem ecotype. Fifty kg of fresh fruits yield 30 kg of seed, which gives about 6 kg of oil and 24 kg of seed cake. Seed viability ranges from 6 to 8 weeks but thoroughly cleaned and properly dried and cooled seeds remain viable upto 6 month. Propagation by stumps and stem cuttings also is practised. Plantlets, produced by tissues cult ring, have also been used for propagation with partial successes.

Azadirachtin, a neem derivative nets Rs. 1.5 lakhs per gram. It is thus essential to establish a elite neem clone, which would increase the returns for a neem tree grower. Identification of a high yielding stain of neem is essential.

The neem tree could practically grow in any type of soil while black soil is most suitable. Studies have indicated that the neem tree actually improves the quality of degraded soil.

Uttar Pradesh has the largest number of Neem trees in the country, a majority of which are on the user lands. Neem tree have higher survival rate than trees of the other species, which indicate a hardiness enabling it to survive even in wasteland. 96 per cent neem trees survived at trail plots, while only 54 per cent and 26 per cent respectively of babul and Sirish tree. These trees, by virtue of their perenial habitat, experience the greatest exposure and are influenced greatly by any appreciable change in the environment.

As regards environmental protection, trees assimilate and accumulate pollutants through the stomas in the leaves and purify the environment, SO_2 sorption in Neem can be more than 14 μg SO_2 sorbed per g fresh weight per hour. Neem and peepal stand out for their SO_2 sink properties.

Chemical Nature of Neem

Neem, a member of the Meliacese family, is a botanical cousin of Mahogany. Neem is bitter in taste. The bitterness is due to the presence of an arry of complex compounds called "Triterpenes" or more specially, "limonoids". More than 100 bioactive compounds, mostly tetranotriterpenoids, diterpenoids, triterpenoids, pentenortriterpenoids, hexanotriterpenoids, and some norterpenoids have been isolated from various parts of the neem tree, still more are being isolated. This formidable array of highly bioactive compounds make neem a unique plant with potential applications in agriculture, public health, and for regulating even human fertility.

The limonoids in neem belong to nine basic structure groups such as *azadırone* (from oil, all four rungs of the basic skeleton intact), *amorastaitin* (from fresh neem leaves), the eco-system related to *gednnin* (from seed oil and bark), *Vepinin* (from seed oil), and *Vilasinin* (from leaves and seed), *nimbolin* (from neem kernel), and *salanin* (from fresh leaves and seed), and the aza group (from neem seed; basically nimbolinin type compounds). Azadirachtin and its analogues have fascinated researchers for the past 30 years because of phagoregellency, growth inhibition and chemosterilizing effects on insects pests. Derivatives of the Neem tree are extensively used in plant protection, as nitrogen-fixers, in human and veterinary medicine and a wide range of toiletries, due to their bio-degradable and non-toxic qualities. Neem cake contains methionine and lysine which are very much required in the poultry feed. Neem leaf extract, neem oil is used to prevent afflatoxicosis in feed and to prevent other infections caused by bacteria.

'Researched' Neem, a Modern Gift

Azadirachta indica A. Duss (neem) is grown throughout the tropics for its multiple utility. In the recent years, neem has created a wide sensation in various countries of the world. The tremendous amount of scientific research being carried out all over the world is wind bogging. Natural Research Council of Washington, D.C., after a lot of painstaking research unambiguously declared Neem as the "Tree for the twenty-first century". In their submission in 1992, they had no hesitation in declaring that "the plant may usher an era in pest control, provide millions with inexpensive medicines, cut down human population growth and even reduce erosion, deforestation and the excessive temperature of an overhead globe.

Traditionally farmers used neem leaves (dried), neem twigs paddles in the field and application of neem cake as fertilisers. Recently, considerable potentialities of Neem as fertiliser has also been reported and neem leaves and cakes have been found to be promising, neem leaves (green) are puddled in flooded rice fields. Dry leaves may be used as much. Neem cake has considerable local potential as fertilisers. It has unique promise as a fertiliser as it contains more nitrogen, phosphorous and potassium, calcium and magnesium than farm yard manure or sewage sluge (Radwanski and Wickens, 1981). In India, it is widely used to fertilise cash crop, particularly sugarcane and vegetable. Oil cake makes soil more fertile due to an ingredient present, which blocks soil bacteria from converting nitrogenous compounds into useless nitrogen gas. When mixed with urea, neem cake cuts down the amount of urea, converted into nitrogen gas in the soil. Use of 'Nimin' coated urea reduces losses of fertiliser nitrogen through leaching and denitrification by 30-35 per cent. In turn, this resulted in improved fertiliser nitrogen utilisation and yield of crop by 25 per cent, depending upon crop and soil types, thus taking major part in nutrients supply and management.

Integrated Nutrient Management and Neem

Integrated nutrient management is defined as the best possible combination of available nutrient management practices, which is biophysically powerful, economically attractive and socially acceptable. The interdisciplinary approach is a necessary response to the fact that farmers goals are not only economic but cultural, social and ecological as well.

During the last two decades, agricultural production has increased in developed and certain developing countries due to use of high yielding varieties and enhanced consumption of chemical fertilisers.

The tremendous increase in plant nutrient consumption indicates the importance of fertilisers to crop production. The extensive and intensive use of organic fertilisers form maximum crop production indirectly leaves residual toxic substances in food which is taken by animals as well as human beings (Gupta and Upadhyay, 1998). The modern day intensive crop cultivation which requires the use of chemical fertilisers are not only in short supply but expensive. Therefore, it is now essential to evolve and adopt a strategy of integrated nutrient supply by using a judicious combination of chemical fertilisers. Organic manures and biofertilisers. Neem cake can make a significant contribution towards the development of strategies for productivity improvement.

Neem and Soil Fertility

Good soil fertility means food crop yield. Traditionally farmers used neem leaves (dried), neem twigs paddled in the field and application of neem cake have been found to be promising; neem leaves (green) are paddled in flooded rice fields and dry leaves may be used as much. Neem cake unique promise as a fertiliser as it contains more nitrogen, phosphorous and potassium, calcium and magnesium than farm yard manure (Radwanski and Wickens, 1981). According to Vyas *et al.*, 1996, laboratory and field trials conducted over seven years have shown that 'Nimin' an neem coated urea reduces losses of fertiliser nitrogen through leaching and denitrification by 30 to 35 per cent. In turn, this resulted in improved fertiliser nitrogen utilisation and increased yield of crop by 25 per cent, depending upon crop and soil type.

Neem cake is the major byproduct of the neem oil crushing industry. It contains 1.07 to 1.36 per cent sulphur and nitrogen content of 2 to 3 per cent. Neem cake is used as manure. Experiments conducted at Kanpur revealed that Neem and castor cakes contains of 7.1 per cent and 4.6 per cent N respectively, mineralised only 61 per cent. Results on the effect of neem cake coating/blending of prilled urea are available from a number of experiments on several crops which reveals that it is an effective way for increasing the crop growth and yield, particularly of the crops grown during rainy season such as rice, cotton, sugarcane and jute. Thus the manurial value of deoiled Neem cake is well established. Neem leaves are used as mulch and manure to increase the soil fertility, as also productivity of crops. Neem plants parts and products used as biofertilisers and important neem chemicals are represented in Fig. 11.1 and Fig. 11.2 respectively.

A large number of field experiments at different locations have clearly demonstrated the advantage of using Nimin, a neem coating urea. The results related to some crops are summarised in Table 11.1 (Vyas, 1996).

Table 11.1: Benefits of Using Nimin Coated Urea in Field Crops

Crops	No. of Trials	% Increase in Yield of the Produce with NCU *vis-a-vis* Uncoated Urea	Cost Benefit Ratio
Rice	65	4.8— 49.7	1 : 2.7—11.4
Wheat	7	6.8— 26.9	1 : 6.0—11.0
Maize	5	17.4— 51.5	1 : 5.8—30.0
Sugarcane	21	4.8— 13.4	1 : 2.8— 6.8
Tea	3	2.4— 2.6	1 : 10.8—12.4
Black pepper	2	26.4—280.0	1 : 3.6—59.4

Source: Summary of Multi-locational Trials, Vyas, 1996.

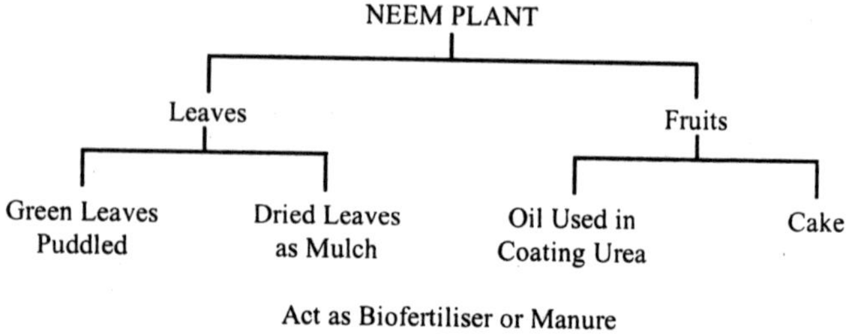

Fig. 11.1: Parts of Neem Plants Used as Biofertiliser

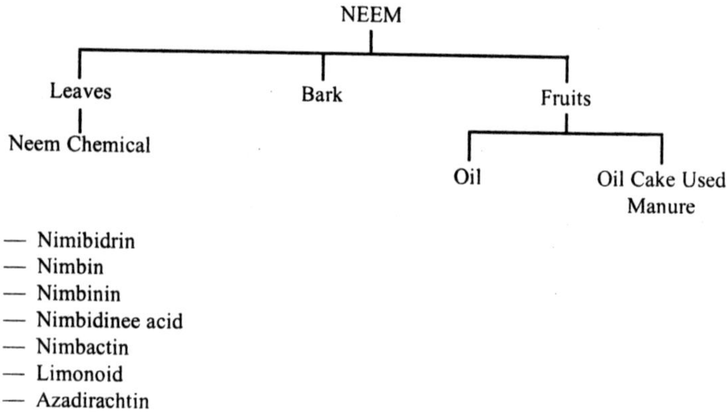

Fig. 11.2: Neem Derivatives Used in Agriculture

It now becomes clear from the data that, marked yield improvement is possible by using 'Nimin' a Neem coated of urea, it is believed that Nimin is responsible for reduction in losses of fertilisers nitrogen. The use of neem products will also be useful with other major fertilisers used namely, diammonium phosphate (DAP), since DAP also contains 18 per cent nitrogen in ammonical form. Effective nutrient management in general, and nitrogen and phosphorus in particular will get a major boost, by using neem products.

The results presented in Table 11.2 indicate that maximum values of dry matter yield, nitrogen uptake and apparent nitrogen recovery were obtained with NCU (Neem Coated Urea) application which is superior to 3 split applications of uncoated urea. For both rice and maize, 70 kg N/ha applied in the form of NCU was at par with 100 kg N/ha applied as uncoated urea.

Table 11.2: Influence of 'Nimin', a Neem Coated Urea on Yield and N Uptake by Rice and Maize Plants under Green House Conditions

Treatments	Dry Matter Yield (g)		Total N Uptake (mg/pot)		Apparent N Recovery (%)	
	Rice	Maize	Rice	Maize	Rice	Maize
1. Control (O-nitrogen)	51.2	47.0	453.6	273.5	—	—
2. Uncoated Urea (100 kg N/ha) single basal application	57.5	56.7	547.1	362.3	34.2	35.5
3. Uncoated Urea (100 kg N/ha) 3 split basal applications	59.4	55.0	596.3	384.4	57.1	44.4
4. Nimim coated urea (100 kg N/ha) single basal applications	66.9	62.8	669.0	414.5	86.1	56.4
5. Nimin coated urea (60 kg N/ha) single basal applications	57.4	56.9	512.6	341.9	39.1	45.6
6. Nimim coated urea (70 kg N/ha) single basal applications	60.3	59.4	544.5	375.6	51.9	58.2
7. Nimin coated urea (80 kg N/ha) single basal application	65.5	58.0	581.6	388.3	64.0	58.4
L.S.D. + (P = 0.05)	4.3	3.8	38.8	30.8	5.4	3.0

Source: Vyas *et al.*, 1991.

$$\text{Apparent N recovery} = \frac{\text{N uptake by plants from N treated plots} - \text{N uptake by plants from control plants}}{\text{N applied plot}} \times 100$$

A large number of field experiments at distant locations were conducted to evaluate the efficiency of 'Nimin' a neem coated urea in rice, wheat, maize, sugarcane and black pepper. The salient findings of these trials are summarised below:

Rice

'Nimin' coated Urea is being evaluated for the three years in the research trials of the All India Council of Agricultural Research. Results obtained from 16 trials at distant location indicated that there was an increase in grain yield of rice ranging from 4.2 to 70.2 per cent in 'Nimin' coated urea plots, as compared to uncoated urea treated plots. On the basis of these trials it was concluded that 'Nimin' coated urea if applied in two split doses performed better in increasing the grain yield and nitrogen use efficiency of rice (Anonymous, 1992).

Wheat and Maize

Two field experiments on wheat during Rabi 1988 and an equal number of trials on maize in Kharif in 1989 demonstrated an increase in the grain yield of 16.7 and 36.9 per cent respectively, in 'Nimin', coated urea treated plots over the plots receiving uncoated urea.

Sugarcane

In a recently concluded study on sugarcane, it was observed that there was a conspicuous increase in the yield with use of 'nimin' coated urea at 100 per cent Nitrogen doses (106.33 t/ha) and 80 per cent Nitrogen (105.6 t/ha) to that over control (75.67 t/ha), prilled urea (98.33 t/ha) and neem cake coated urea (97.3 t/ha).

In this study as well as in earlier studies conducted at the farm of Nizam Sugar Factory Nizamabad, Cauvery Sugar and Chemicals Ltd., Pettaivaytalai and EID Parry, Tamil Nadu; it was found that value of Beix, pot and CCS were higher in 'Nimin', coated urea treated plots than in plots treated with uncoated urea. In a recently concluded study at the research farm of Anakapalle of Andhra Pradesh Agricultural University, 'Nimin', coated urea resulted in increased cane yield by 18.34 per cent in comparison to uncoated urea (Vyas, 1993).

Plantation Crops

Results of field experiments at the experimental farm of the National Research Centre for Spices, Calicut indicated that the application of 'Nimin', coated urea at 100 g/Vine, increased the yield of black pepper by 280 per cent compared to uncoated urea (Vyas, 1993).

The Insight of Role of Neem Products in Enhanced Used Efficiency

Preventing the loss of plant nutrients from an eco-system is important for soil fertility management. Nitrogen, phosphorus and potassium (N, P, K) are the three major elements which determine soil fertility and should be ideally present in 4 : 2 : 1 ratio; aberrations affect fertility and thus crop yield. Urea containing 48 per cent of N is applied to crops in the largest amounts; but only less than half of this N, in the form of nitrate is available to the crops. The rest is lost through leaching or by volatilisation or by surface run-off after a heavy shower (Prasad and Power, 1995). Leaching of soluble nitrates into the sub-soil, and eventually into the ground water is well known. Nitrate losses of 50-70 per cent through leaching were observed in rice crops in India. Leaching not only depletes precious nitrate but also takes away clay, soil and organic matter leading to low chemical soil fertility and low plant available plant nutrients reserves. Ammonia volatilisation also can contribute to nearly 60 per cent nitrate loss. Loss through volatilisation occurs when the denitrifying bacteria reduces the nitrate elemental nitrogen and nitrous oxide which escape to the statosphere and cause ozone depletion and also thus contribute to greenhouses warming. On the other hand, nitrate build up in drinking water can reduce the blood's ability to transport oxygen, especially if the nitrates are converted to nitrites ('blue-baby syndrome'). Even ruminants are vulnerable to, nitrate nitrite poisoning leading to poor growth rates, reduce milk production, and increased susceptibility to infections and even abortions.

Excellent work has been done by C. Dev Kumar *et al.* (1985) in identifying the compounds in Neem extracts which are responsible for nitrification inhibition. In the similar line Bains *et al.* (1971) in field trials found an excellent nitrification inhibitor, even better than sulphur coated urea. Ammonia volatilisation, urea hydrolysis and leaching, were all reduced when urea was blended or coated with neem cake. Results from several field experiments show that neem cake coating or prilled urea increased nitrogen uptake by 4.5 to 19.4 per cent. The increase in rice yield due to neem cake coating/blending of prilled urea ranged from 1 to 54 per cent, the average being 9.6 per cent. Neem cake coated urea applied to rice or sugarcane increased yield by 7 per cent in the ratoon sugarcane (Sharma *et al.*, 1981). Ready to use 'Nimin' (containing 5 per cent neem bitter tertranortriterpenoids) are now commercially available. Application of Nimin coated urea (1 part Nimin: 100 part urea wt wt-1) reduced losses of fertiliser N through leaching and denitrification by 30-35 per cent and increased yields in treated crops upto 25 per cent (Vyas *et al.*, 1996). The bitter in Nimin delay the denitrification process up to 30 days either killing nitrifying bacteria or suppressing their activity. Coating urea with Nimin could bring a saving 20 per cent of urea. The technology is becoming popular with farmers in India where annual Nimin sales are now ca. 700 metric tons.

Nimin for Enhanced Use Efficiency

Nimin coated urea was examined for hydrolytic degration as well as nitrification in two different soils types, namely a laterite (Ultisol) and a medium black (Vertisol) at two moisture regions upland as well as flooded. The data on the nitrite and nitrate nitrogen content in both the soil and water regions increase upto a period of one month when soils were treated with Nimin coated urea.

In contrast, a sharp increase in nitrite and nitrate nitrogen levels within a period of 7 or 15 days was observed in soils treated with uncoated urea. The values of nitrite and nitrate nitrogen were used to calculate per cent nitrification inhibition in soil and these values are reported in Table 11.3. The data clearly indicate a significant inhibition of nitrification in Nimin coated urea treated soils at least for 30 days. Further, the data on ammonical nitrogen content did not reveal any notable difference between the rate of hydrolysis of two urea forms.

Table 11.3: Influence of Nimin Coated Urea (NCU) on Nitrification Inhibition (NI) in Two Soils under Moisture Regimes

	Per cent Nitrification Inhibition Days after incubation			
	3	7	15	30
Laterite Soil				
Upland conditions	74.4	63.5	53.3	46.2
Flooded conditions	22.1	53.7	25.2	10.5
Black Soil				
Upland conditions	86.9	78.9	57.6	39.7
Flooded conditions	30.1	66.9	36.6	38.8

Source: Vyas *et al.*, 1991.

$$\% \text{ NI} = 100 \times \frac{(NO_2 + NO_3 - \text{N in Urea Treated Soil}) - (NO_2 + NO_3 - \text{N in NCU Treated Soil})}{(NO_2 + NO_3 - \text{N in Urea Treated Soils})}$$

Conclusion

In the recent years, Neem has created a wide sensation in advance countries of the world also. This plant is proved beneficial for agricultural fertiliser management programme specially for the nitrogenous fertilisers, and helpful in minimising the adverse impact of nitrogenous fertilisers to human health and environment. The constituents from neem seed when coated with urea have been found to very effective in slowing down the rate of nitrification. This has resulted in reducing upto 35 per cent in urea consumption and /or increase upto 9 per cent in the yield of various agri-crops. Enough work has been done over the last several years through Indian Council of Agricultural Research (ICAR), at its various research stations and also through agricultural Universities to confirm these fact.

REFERENCES

Anonymous (1992). *Neem—A tree for Solving Global Problems*. Report of an adhoc panel of the board on Science and Technology for International Academy Press.

Bains, S.S.; Prasad, R. and Bhatia, P. (1971). "Use of Indigenous Materials to Enhance the Efficiency of Fertilizer Nitrogen for Rice", *Fertile. News*, 16 (3): 30-32.

Deva Kumar, C.; Goswami, B.K. and Mukherjee, S.K. (1985). "Nematicidal Principles from Neem (*Azadirachta Indica* A. Juss. I.). Screening Neem Fraction against *Meloidogyne incognita*", *Indian Journal of Nematology*, 15 (1): 121-124.

Gupta, R.C. and Upadhyay, D.N. (1998). Neem in Applied Human Ecology and Sustainable Development in Neem: *Application in Agriculture, Health Care and Environment*, (ed.) B. Venketeshwarlu.

Prasad, R. and Power, J.F. (1995). "Nitrification Inhibitors for Agriculture, Health and the Environment", *Adv. in Sgeon.*, 54: 233-281.

Radwanski, S.A. and Wickens, G.E. (1981). "Vegetative Fellow and Potential Value of the Neem Tree (Azadirachta indica) in the Tropics", *Econ. Bot.*, 35: 398-414.

Sharma, S.N.; Singh, S.; Sharma, R.P.; Parashar, K.S. and Prasad, R. (1981). "Studies on Carry-over Effects of Urea, Sulfur Coated Urea, Neem Cake Coated Urea and Nitrapyrin Treated Urea Applied to Plant Sugarcane Crop on the Succeeding Ratoon—A Acker Planzenbau", *J. Agron. Crop. Sci.*, 150: 207-214.

Vyas, B.N. (1993). *Coating of Urea Fertilizer for Enhanced Use Efficiency and Environment Protection: Process and Plant Engineering*, 129-132.

Vyas, B.N. (1996). Role of Neem Compounds in Improving Fertilizer Use Efficiency and Pest Control: *In Neem: Applications in Agriculture, Health Care and Environment*, (ed.) B. Venketeshwarlu.

Vyas, B.N.; Wodreg, N.B. and Mistry, K.B. (1991). "Development and Evaluation of Neem Extract as a Coating for Urea Fertilizer", *Fertilizer News*, 19-25.

Vyas, B.N.; Wodreg, N.B. and Highway, K.B. (1996). *Potential of Nimim-Coated Urea for Enhancing Nitrogen Efficiency by Crops*, Paper presented at Int. Neem Conf., Australia, 1996 (abstract).

12

BALANCED USE OF FERTILISERS
Before and After Decontrol

— *V.J. Bhave*

India has primarily been an agrarian economy with 65 per cent of its workforce engaged in agriculture and allied operations. Self-sufficiency in food has been the guiding principle of Indian agricultural policy since independence. Agriculture is also the source of supply of raw materials to industries like cotton and jute textiles, sugar, rubber, etc. Much of the small scale sector like handloom weaving, oil crushing, rice husking, etc. is dependent on agriculture for its raw material. Together, they account for 50 per cent of the income generated in the manufacturing sector. Importance of agriculture also arises from the role it plays in India's trade. Products like tea, sugar, oilseeds, tobacco, spices, constitute a major chunk of India's exports.

Indian agriculture is characterised by overdependence on uncertain rains, multiplicity of crops, dominance of small and marginal farmers, etc. All these result in the agricultural productivity being low.

The Indian population is expected to reach 1 billion mark by 2000 AD. The Planning Commission has indicated that 240 million MTS of foodgrains would have to be produced in order to feed this population.

There are three factors that are involved in the increase in agricultural production. These are: (i) increase in area under crops, (ii) improvement in cropping patterns, (iii) improvement in productivity per hectare.

Due to the fast growing population and rapid urbanisation, the area under crops has remained more or less constant. The climatic and socio-economic diversity of the Indian crop production scene is replete with different cropping patterns. Socio economically, the peasantry ranges from subsistence farmers to affluent farmers who operate with a high input intensity in agriculture.

Fertilisers have been considered to be the kingpin in the process of agricultural production. Their judicious use in the right combination and in the right type of soil for the appropriate crop is a prerequisite to an efficient agricultural production strategy. For every tonne of fertiliser nutrient put into the soil, there is an increase of 8 to 10 tonnes of foodgrains, other things remaining equal. It has been estimated that about 70 per cent of the growth in agricultural production can be attributed to increased fertiliser use.

Recognising the importance of fertilisers in boosting agricultural production, the Government of India had controlled the pricing and distribution of fertilisers under the Essential Commodities Act, 1956. No company could market its entire production in any one state and nor was any state dependent only on one manufacturer for its supply of fertilisers. To increase fertiliser consumption which was at a low 0.55 kg. per hectare in 1951-52, the Government pegged the prices at a level affordable to the farmer, which was, in most cases, lower than the costs of production. It took almost 40 years for the level to come upto 70 kg of nutrients per hectare, which is still, far below the levels used in developed countries.

As a part of the liberalisation process, the Government of India decontrolled phosphatic and potassic fertilisers in August 1992. This resulted in a doubling of the selling prices of these fertilisers which sent the consumption of P & K down from 33.2 lakh MTS and 13.6 lakh MTS of P & K respectively (1991-92) to 28.43 lakh MTS(P) and 8.84 lakh MTS (K) in 1992-93. On the other hand, N consumption increased from 80.5 lakh MTS to 84.3 lakh MTS in the same period.

Not only has consumption of P and K fallen, but this has adversely affected the fertiliser industry which manufactures these products in terms of reduced capacity utilisation, high costs, etc.

While application of fertiliser nutrients is essential for a high crop yield, the fertilisers need to be applied in proper proportion to each other. Any imbalance in this would have a long term effect on soil fertility. The NPK ratio in 1991-92 was 5.9 : 2.4 : 1 which was distorted by the decontrol to 9.5 : 3.2 : 1 in 1992-93.

While increased use of nitrogen may result in plant growth reduction in P and K would delay the maturity of seeds and fruits and weaken the plants.

The resistance to adequate use of P and K by the farmers has come primarily because of the high prices. N continues to be used as before because of the controlled and low price of urea which is a nitrogenous fertiliser.

To partially absorb the shock of high prices, the Government introduced an adhoc subsidy scheme for phosphatic and potassic fertilisers ranging from Rs. 340 to Rs. 1000 PMT.

Concern has been expressed by the fertiliser industry as well as agricultural universities and other experts that the continued distortion in application ratios of fertilisers may damage soil fertility for a long time.

One of the options suggested to remedy the situation is to increase prices of urea in a phased manner so as to bring it in line with the relative prices of phosphatic and potassic fertilisers.

However, the immediate task is to convince the farmers of the importance of balanced use of fertilisers for higher productivity. This can be accomplished through focused campaigns by the industry, agricultural universities, State/Central Government, and other agencies.

Along with tremendous publicity, fertiliser promotion campaigns with the same theme need to be implemented across the country. Especially, the use of tools like demonstrations, would bring about far reaching effects in the area of balanced fertilisation. Farmer contact programmes need to stress this aspect. Manufacturers, in addition to promoting their own brands, need to extend their objectives to incorporate this theme in their activities. For, so long as the farmer survives, the industry survives, and on the survival of the industry rests the future of India.

13

FERTILISER USE EFFICIENCY UNDER DECONTROLLED SCENARIO

— A.K. Kar

In 1992, Government took major policy decisions first to decanalise some of the raw materials like Rock Phosphate, Ammonia, etc. used in the manufacture of phosphatic fertilisers and then to decontrol the pricing, distribution and movement of phosphatic and potassic fertilisers, keeping Urea under the control of Retention Pricing Scheme. As a result of these decisions, the prices of phosphate and potash had more than doubled and that of urea remained almost same. The overall impact can be summarised as follows:

(*Million tons*)

	1992-92	1994-95
N	8.00	9.50
P	3.30	2.90
K	1.36	1.06
NPK Ratio	5.9 : 2.4 : 1	8.9 : 2.8 : 1

The declining ratio in the use of NPK has created an alarming situation in the maintenance of soil fertility. Under this situation, the basic objective should be to increase the consumption of phosphate and potash, at the same time maintain the current growth trend in the use of nitrogen to attain the ideal NPK ratio of 4 : 2 : 1. With the steep increase in the prices of phosphate and potash, more attention should be given on fertiliser use efficiency, so that the farmers may derive maximum benefit out of every rupee spent on fertilisers. This calls for better understanding of some basic factors of nutrient management in soil.

Nitrogen Management

The major sources of nitrogen in soil are organic matter like crop residues, farm manure, legumes and fertiliser. Organic matter on decomposition releases nitrogen in available ammonium and nitrate forms.

Decomposition of Organic Matter

$$\begin{array}{c}\text{Organic Matter}\\ +\\ \text{Moist Warm Soil}\end{array} \xrightarrow[\text{attack}]{\text{Microbial}} \begin{array}{l}\text{(i) Easily decomp. compds.}\\ \\ \text{(ii) Resistant compds. like fats, oils, lignins.}\end{array}$$

Organic matter on decomposition releases nutrients like nitrogen, phosphorus, potassium, calcium, mangnesium, sulphur and micro-nutrients slowly in easily available form depending on soil moisture, pH, temperature, etc.

(i) $\text{(C, H. Containing) compds.} + O_2 \xrightarrow[\text{oxidation}]{\text{Enzymic}} CO_2 + H_2O + \text{Energy}$

> ½ *of dry wt.*

(ii) $\text{Proteins R–NH}_2 \xrightarrow[\text{hydrolysis (bacterias, fungi, actionomycetis)}]{\text{Enzymic}} NH_4 \xrightarrow[\text{oxidation}]{\text{+ Enzymic}} NO_2^- + H^+ \longrightarrow$

$NO_3^- + \text{Energy}$

(a) In absence of Oxygen as in the case of flooded rice soil, the decomposition of protein stops at NH_4^+ stage, so most of the available nitrogen in rice soil is in NH_4^+ form.

(b) Nitrification results in an increase in soil acidity. This effect is of more significance in case of fertilisers containing ammonium salts.

(c) Application of organic matter in pre-Kharif season gives better results than application in cooler Rabi season.

(d) Nitrogenous fertilisers should not be applied within 15 days of application of green organic matter/undecomposed organic matter in soil to check immobilisation of nitrogen.

(e) Composting is a must to derive the maximum benefit from all the organic waste products.

Fate of N-fertilisers in Soil

	% of Fertiliser N	
	Average	Range
(i) Crop removal	60	25—70
(ii) Added to organic matter reserve and mineralised subsequently	15	0—40
(iii) Leaching	5	0—60
(iv) Volatilisation as ammonia	5	0—50
(v) Denitrification	15	0—40

(a) N-fertiliser is soluble in moisture and very mobile in soil. Nitrogen is very susceptible to losses through gaseous transformation, run off, leaching, etc.

(b) Since our primary objective of fertiliser application is to maximise the crop removal of nutrients, attention should be given to the choice of right kind of fertilisers, placement technique and timing of application.

(c) The magnitude of crop response to applied N depends on number of factors—type of crop variety, the rate of application standard of agronomic practices followed and other factors.

(d) Nutrient removal studies have shown that per ton of rice grain production 20 kg N and wheat grain, 30 kg N is required.

Phosphorus Management

Phosphorus in plant system enhances early root growth and root matrix formation that helps in removal of nutrients from soil more efficiently. Later on during reproductive phase phosphorus initiates flowering, fruiting and grain formation.

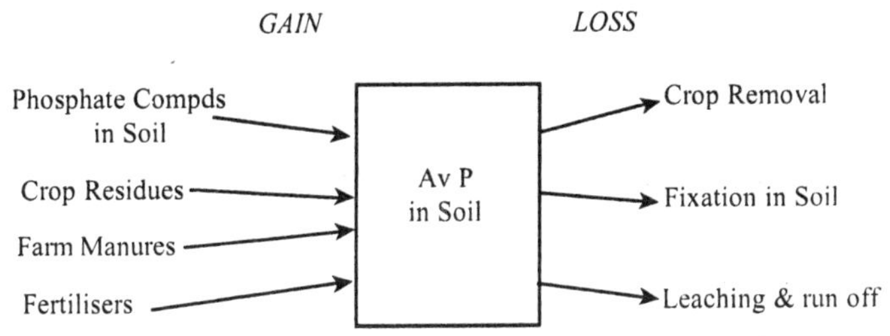

(i) The removal of P by growing plants is comparatively less than that of N and K. Consequently the loss of P through crop removal is *not much* nor is the return of P in Crop residues of major importance. Because of the relative insolubility of soil phosphorus compounds and the less mobility of phosphates, the leaching of P is essentially *nil*.

(ii) The amount of available phosphorus in the soil at any one time is relatively small compared to that of Ca, Mg, K, etc. The availability of P is largely determined by (a) Soil pH; (b) soluble Fe, Al, Mn; (c) presence of Fe, Al, Mn containing minerals; (d) available Ca; and (e) amount and decomposition of organic matter.

(iii) The overall phosphorus problem is three-fold—(a) to increase the release of native P; (b) addition of P fertilisers; (c) regulation of the fixation of added P in soil through the right choice of P-fertilisers as per soil conditions.

(iv) Judicious liming practices to maintain the soil pH between 6-7 results in release of native P and minimise the fixation of added P.

(v) A top dressing of P fertiliser within 3 weeks after sowing/planting gives higher yield.

Fate of P-Fertilisers

	% of Fertiliser P	
	Average	Range
Crop removal (3 reap period)	20	5—30
Held in Soil	80	60—95
Leaching & Run off	< 2	0—10
	100	

In soil of pH 6-7, water soluble phosphate fertilisers like super phosphate, DAP, etc. gives good response but in acid soils partially citrate soluble fertiliser like Suphala is preferred due to less fixation. In plantation crops part of the P dose may be applied as grounded rock phosphate.

Potassium Management

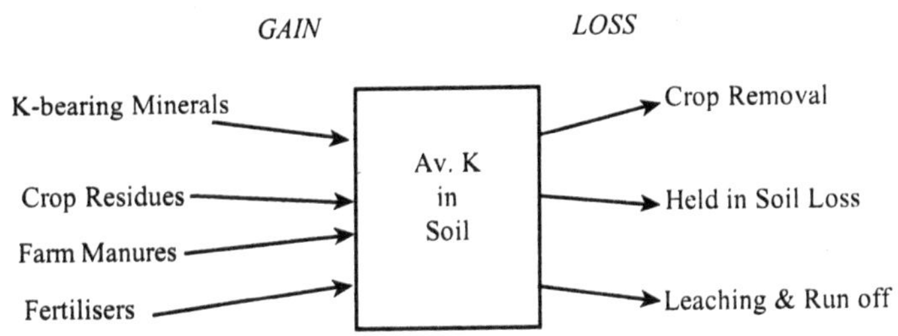

(i) Most soil contains large store of potassium through the K-bearing minerals like mica, feldspars, etc. The total and exchangeable K will be more if illite is the dominant clay mineral in soil.

(ii) Crop removal of K generally exceeds that of the other essential elements. Hence the return of Crop residues and manures is very important in maintaining soil potash.

(iii) A considerable amount of K is also fixed within the layer lattice of expanding type of clay minerals like montmerillanite.

(iv) Though our soils are fairly rich in K, in intensive cropping areas, balanced K-fertiliser should be applied.

(v) Top dressing of K, especially in light soils gives better yield.

Fate of K-fertilisers

	% of Fertiliser P	
	Average	Range
Crop removal	80—85	50—100
Held in soil	15	0—50
Leaching & run off	< 5	0—10
	100	

Nutrients—Method of Reaching Root Surface

Plant root absorb nutrients through root interception, mass flow of nutrients by movement of soil moisture and diffusion of nutrients to the root surface. Plant roots occupy only about 1-2 per cent of the soil volume.

(% contribution)

Nutrient	Root Interception	Mass Flow	Diffusion
N	1	99	0
P	3	6	91
K	2	17	81

The importance of water flow in the availability of nutrients, especially nitrogen is revealed from the above Table. A considerable amount of soluble N remains within root zone for considerable periods without being absorbed and used by plants—depending on (i) water movement, (ii) root flux and root activity. Only 50-60 per cent of the water held at field capacity is available to crops, hence only 50-60 per cent of the N could be brought to the plant roots and get absorbed inside the plants. Water have to be replenished a number of times to carry larger proportion of N to plants.

It can also be noted that availability of Phosphorus and Potassium is rather independent of moisture status in soil.

14

DISTRIBUTION OF FERTILISER UPTO FARMERS LEVEL AND LEGAL ASPECTS OF FERTILISER
A Panel Discussion

— *S.S. Anand*

Fertiliser manufacturers spend a considerable time and energy while selecting the distribution channel. At the present era of marketing scenario there is a need for rationalisation of distributional and movement of decontrolled fertilisers with a view to reduce the selling price to the farmers on the one hand and sustain the availability of the products on the other. For this, proper management of warehousing and handling specifically the rationalisation of the location, size, number of warehouses and minimisation of number of handlings, could help in reducing the marketing costs. Detailed micro level planning was an essential input to ensure the success of the efforts in the distribution channel. The distribution channel is very much dependent on production and consumption. In 1994-95, the total production and consumption in India was as follows:

Table 14.1: The Total Production and Consumption of Fertiliser in 1994-95

(In lakh tonnes)

	Production	Consumption
N	79.44	95.11
P_2O_5	25.57	29.44
K_2O	Import (12.82)	10.64

The agricultural inputs reached the farmers through different marketing channels and operative systems through over 2,30,000 retail outlets. The major distribution system of fertiliser is through private sector and cooperative sector.

Besides this, State Agro Industries Corporation and own Service Centres of manufacturers are also there. From manufacturers movement of fertilisers is restricted through wholesaler and wholesaler to dealer and from dealer to farmers. In cooperative, other hand from manufacturer to State Marketing Federation to district level cooperatives to primary cooperative societies and ultimately it goes to the farmers.

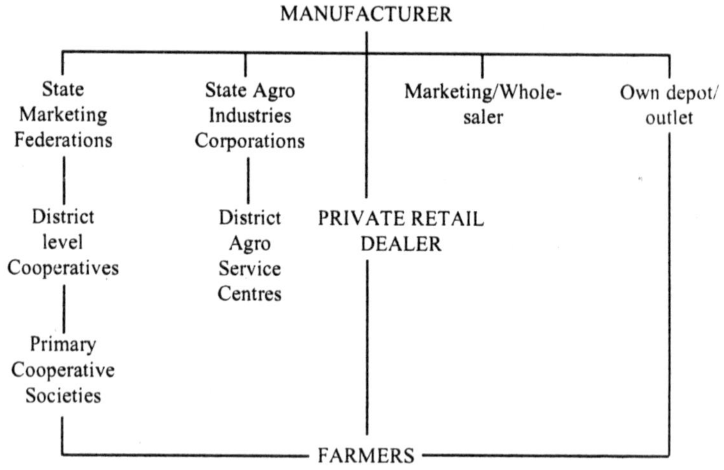

Legal Aspects

Legal aspects of fertiliser marketing starting from production of fertiliser till it reaches to the hand of farmers, different steps are involved for distribution of fertiliser to the farmers.

(a) *Issue of Licence:* This provides the charging of fees as a specified in the order against issue of licence. Each institution/private dealer etc. dealing with fertiliser should have fertiliser licence duly obtained from competent authority (State Government).

(b) *E.C.A.:* The price of the fertiliser has been regulated under sub-sections 3(2) (c), 2(d) of the same section empowers for regulating the issue of licences, permits, storage, transport, distribution, disposal, acquisition use or consumption of the fertiliser. It also provides for the production of books of accounts, records relating to their business and to furnish such information relating thereto.

The Central Government may with a view to regulating equitable distribution of fertilisers and making fertilisers available at fair prices, by notification in the official gazette, fixes the maximum price or rates at which any fertiliser may be sold by dealer, manufacturer, importer or pool handling agency.

Display of stock position and price list of fertilisers—Every dealer who makes or offers to make a retail sale of any fertilisers shall permanently display in his place of business.

Issue of Cash/Credit memorandum—Every dealer shall issue a cash or credit memorandum to a purchaser of a fertiliser in the Form 'M'.

Dealers to be registered—No person, including manufacturer, importer, pool handling agency, a wholesaler dealer, a retail dealer etc. shall offer for sale of fertilisers at any place except in accordance with the terms and conditions of the certificate of registration granted to him.

Source Certificate

For distribution or calling out fertiliser business by the dealer or retailer, they should have the source certificate. Different sources of service are requested for selling fertilisers from different sources. The source of certificate should be in the Form 'O'. For the renewal of the certificate, the holder of the certificate has to apply in the Form 'C' in duplicate together with the prescribed fee and source of certificate. If the application is made after the expiry of the date, but within 30 days from the date of expiry, additional fee as prescribed by the State Government has to be paid.

Quality control is a major aspect in legal aspect of fertiliser marketing. For quality control of fertiliser, each grade should have as per specifications of F.C.O. *e.g.*, for Urea:

(i) Moisture—per cent by weight maximum—1.0
(ii) Total Nitrogen, per cent by weight minimum—46
(iii) Biuret, per cent by weight maximum—1.5
(iv) Particle size—90 per cent of the materials shall passed through 4 mm. I.S. Sieve etc.

Legal aspect in respect of the transportation logistic—This should be either through Rail movement or Road movement. Specific freight charges and challan for Road movement should be with them.

It is also specified that commodities which are likely to undergo significant variation in weight or measure on account of environmental or other conditions may be qualified by the words when packed and when such qualification is made the package containing such commodity shall also been thereon information with regard to the matter specified nutrient content, gross content, net content in a package containing fertiliser should be there.

Samples—Different types of samples are available in the market and the best suited is to be taken to draw the sample as per procedure given in the F.C.O.

For better distribution and to keep the image of the manufacturer, a constant vigilance for the quality control is necessary right from the production level to the distribution system at retailers point. For this purpose, preventive measures should have to be taken.

15

FERTILISER USE IN MAJOR FIELD CROPS IN NAGALAND

— *S. Yehoto Ayemi* and *N.P. Singh*

Agriculture and Socio-Economic Background

The State is still reeling under subsistence Agriculture and our economy is predominantly agrarian. Food production is not even enough for the families or State population. The impact of the technology is very low and tribal and clan connections are very strong.

Land holdings are fragmented. More than 50 per cent of land holders have more than 10 ha of land but fragmented.

Farming system is not economical and integrated. Our farmers follow mostly monoculture of paddy crop which is a low value crop. Double cropping/multicropping is almost absent. Shifting cultivation predominates. Land available for mechanisation in the foothills is not much and not properly reclaimed. The fertiliser consumption is very low (6 kg/ha in 94-95).

Actual land tillers are becoming lesser and lesser. As per 1991 census report, only 30.71 per cent of the people work in the cultivation activities and that too only few months. Non-farming activities during the off-season are not available to raise the income of the farmers. Many school dropouts are staying in the villages as parasites to the parents and shuttle between the village and towns without any jobs.

Area under irrigation is shown around 66,000 ha but this is also rainfed and can hardly support one crop of paddy.

Nearly 90 per cent of the land is under hilly terrain and because of this productivity is low and prone to heavy soil erosion.

Degree of deforestation is very fast and the forest resources have dwindled considerably. The process have become irreversible now.

Potential markets for our agricultural produce are located far off and also the marketing network is not organised properly.

When we see the trend of the growth of our population, it is expanding rapidly, say from 7.75 lakhs in 1971 to 12.09 lakhs in 1991. The projection in 1996 is about 15.14 lakhs and in 2000 A.D. is going to be 18.15 lakhs respectively. It can be assumed that the population is going to be double at the interval of 25 years (1971-1996).

Table 15.1: Area and Production under Major Crops (1994-95)

Sl. No.	Crops	Area (ha)	Production (M.T.)
1.	Rice	1,36,000	1,74,000
2.	Maize	27,000	28,000
3.	Pulses	6,000	4,000
4.	Oilseeds	7,000	6,800
5.	Potato	4,500	29,000
	Total	1,80,500	2,42,000

The present level of productivity of food crops in Nagaland is 1.22 M.T. per ha which is far below the National average. The only way to increase the productivity will be mainly through the use of fertilisers. Long term fertiliser experiments conducted in India and elsewhere in the world have clearly brought out the fact that balanced use of plant nutrients is important to sustain crop productivity and soil fertility. Omission of any plant nutrient required by crop would certainly have deleterious effect on crop yield and its quality. The imbalanced application of nutrients is going to have adverse effect on their yields on long term basis including profitability to the farmers.

Considering the nutrient removal by crops and supply through different sources of plant nutrients, including fertilisers, it is seen that removal is far greater than the supply. As a result, soils are being consistently mined. With the present trend in soil nutrient replenishment, it would not be possible to increase yield level, rather a decline would be noticed shortly, unless balanced fertilisers are applied adequately.

To supplement inorganic fertilisers, biofertilisers can also be used for increasing productivity level and also to maintain the soil health.

Trend in the Consumption of Fertiliser

The consumption of fertiliser is on the increasing trend. The official figure may show arratic trend because the procurement by the department is dependent on the fund available for purchase of fertiliser for subsidy sale. But the sale through the private dealers especially Dimapur area seems to be bulky.

Table 15.2: Mean Fertility Status of Soils of Nagaland by Blocks

Name of the Block	Analysis				Rating		
	pH	Org. C.	Av. Phosphate in kg/ha	Av. Potash in kg/ha	Nitrogen	Phosphate	Potash
1. Ghaspani	6.32	1.160	41.7	592.0	H	L	M
2. Kikruma	6.27	2.690	40.0	135.0	H	L	VL
3. Kohima	5.74	1.464	58.0	153.0	H	M	VL
4. Rengma/pughoboto (Tseminyu)	6.00	1.883	100.0	87.5	H	M	VL
5. Chakhesang TD (Phek)	6.83	2.627	113.5	97.9	H	M	H
6. Peren	6.01	2.630	53.7	537.5	H	M	M
7. Changtongyia	5.61	1.333	35.5	385.2	H	L	M
8. Zunheboto	5.73	2.403	46.0	402.7	H	L	M
9. Mongkolemba	5.83	0.958	16.2	400.5	H	VL	M
10. Ongpangkong	5.66	1.535	24.4	537.5	H	VL	M
11. Tokiye	5.93	1.928	76.6	305.2	H	M	L
12. Wakching	5.85	1.778	25.0	103.1	H	VL	VL
13. Mon	5.90	1.10	114.0	68.7	H	M	VL
14. Noklak	5.70	2.683	135.0	125.0	H	H	VL
15. Longleng	6.30	2.376	45.0	1093.7	H	L	H
16. Sangsangyu	5.83	2.038	115.0	652.5	H	M	M
17. Longkhim	5.68	2.943	50.0	604.0	H	L	M

H = High; M = Medium; L = Low; VL = Very low.

Source: Soil Survey Report (1975), Nagaland: Directorate of Agriculture, Nagaland, Kohima.

Table 15.3: Fertiliser Schedule for Crops

Index	Paddy (transplanted)			Ptato			Maize		
	N	P	K	N	P	K	N	P	K
Very low	10C	90	50	100	100	75	87	87	50
Low	75	90	37	87	90	50	75	75	37
Medium	50	50	—	62	70	25	50	50	—
High	37	37	—	50	40	—	37	37	—

The farmers do not apply balanced fertilisers and the ratios are wide among the different crops, e.g. Potato growers apply only D.A.P. and here the ratio is near about 1 : 3 : 0 which is quite imbalanced. Extension workers have to correct this practice by motivating them to mix other fertilisers also. Making the formulated mixed fertilisers available to the farmers may correct the imbalanced use of fertiliser to a great extent.

Fertiliser consumption is not evenly distributed and the commentation is high in places in and around Dimapur and Kohima and is attributable to easy accessibility to the commodity and technology. More demonstration on fertiliser application are required in the less consumption area by both the Department and the FAI.

There are two categories of consumers:

(a) Those who can afford the 50 per cent subsidised rates and their demands are high, e.g. Potato growers for DAP.

(b) Those who can not afford to buy even the subsidised fertiliser, e.g. Rice farmers for DAP and Urea. Price hike on fertilisers has greatly affected our farmers. More price incentive schemes are desired for pushing the fertiliser consumption up. Even if we consider the irrigated area alone, assessment of fertiliser required for Paddy crop in 66,000 ha area it works out to be 6,000 M.T. of Urea, 10,000 M.T. of DAP and 4,000 M.T. of MOP. The financial requirement for procurement of this fertilisers roughly comes to Rs. 1390 lakhs, which is impossible to meet from the annual fund allocation against fertiliser procurement.

The fertiliser use in plantation agriculture is on the rise. Potato and Paddy are the leading crops in order of the fertiliser consumption.

Concluding Remarks

One way to increase the fertiliser consumption in the State is by raising the level of fertiliser consumption in the lesser consuming districts through Fertilisers Demonstrations in farmer's field. For this FAI may associate more actively with the State Department of Agriculture in conducting such Demonstrations/Training in the interior districts.

The consumption can also be increased all over the State by increasing the Central assistance to the North East States for transport/ Fertiliser subsidies.

The experts present in the Seminar specially the extension expert from the FAI may advise/suggest the ways and means to improve the fertiliser consumption level and also on the procurement/marketing of the fertilisers.

Since the subsidised fertiliser cannot meet the demand of the farmers, procurement of bulk fertiliser by the department through the help of credit from some institutions may also be considered in this Seminar.

Paddy farmers in the State complaint about the formation of the hard pan following the application of DAP. This may also be discussed.

Application of common salt in the jhum paddy is commonly practiced in some districts for weed control and the reports have been received that application of this has given better growth and high yield. This may also be discussed whether this will bring adverse effect to the soil health.

16

PRESENT STATUS OF INTEGRATED NUTRIENT SUPPLY MANAGEMENT SYSTEM IN NAGALAND STATE

— *Dipak Chetri*

Geographical and Climatic Features

The State of Nagaland is located in the North-Eastern region of India. It is 16,579 sq km in area, and lies between 90°20′ to 95°15′E longitude and 25°6′ latitude, bordering Myanmar on the East, Manipur on the South, Assam on the West and Arunachal Pradesh on the North.

The State is hilly except a narrow belt of foothills bordering Assam and small valleys in between the lower ranges on the western and north-eastern flanks. The altitude varies from 200 to 3840 metres msl. topographically the landscape can be grouped into three divisions, viz.:

(i) The foothills with undulating to rolling topography and having sub-tropical climate.
(ii) The lower ranges and mid-slopes with varying degrees of slopes and having sub-montane climate.
(iii) High hills and mountainous region above 900 M altitude.

The climate over the foothills is warm sub-tropical and that over the high hills is cool and temperate. The summer and winter temperature over the hills vary from 5°C to 25°C and those over foothills have a range between 12°C to 32°C. The average annual rainfall is between 200 to 250 cms., occurring over about seven months from April to October.

Population

The total population as per the Census of 1991, is 1.22 millions. The present population may be around 1.5 millions, 82 per cent of which live in villages.

Agricultural Scenario in the State

The main food grain crops grown are rice, hill millets, jobstears and maize of which rice is the main staple food of most of the Nagas. The majority of the villagers subsist on slash-and-burn cultivation locally known as Jhum cultivation. The most of the area is under Jhum cultivation. The net area under Jhum cultivation will be about 1.3 lakh hectares. The estimated irrigation potential is 1.80 lakh ha of which 60,000 ha have been developed (1991), most of which is in foot-hill area and is almost rainfed in nature.

Area of production of rice during 1995-96 to 1997-98 in the State is given in Table 16.1.

Table 16.1: Area and Production of Rice during 1995-96 to 1997-98 in the State

	1995-96	1996-97	1997-98
Area ('000 ha)	140.00	140.00	145.00
Production ('000 M.T.)	180.00	153.00	187.00

From the above figure it can be seen that the productivity is very low which is even below 15 quintals per ha.

Prospect of Integrated Nutrient Supply Management System

The farmers of the state hardly use any chemical fertilisers except in few pockets in the crop production programme. As major portion of cropped area is under Jhum, where no visible effect can be expected due to ready run-off loss of applied fertilisers. In the valley areas the farmers are satisfied with the production they get out of using their traditional seed varieties. It has been observed that the farmers in those areas can harvest much more yield out of the HYV seeds supplied by the agriculture department even without using chemical fertilisers. This shows that the soil fertility level in those areas are maintained due to deposition of organic matter through surface run-off from the surrounding hill areas.

The state department of agriculture is advocating farmers to use chemical fertilisers along with organic manures and biofertilisers so as to sustain productivity of land.

Chemical Fertilisers

The average consumption of fertiliser in the state is very much low compared to the national average. The agriculture department is encouraging farmers to use more fertilisers in the crop production programme. For this field demonstrations are conducted on use of fertilisers in various crops.

The fertiliser consumption in the State for last three years are given in Table 16.2.

Table 16.2: Fertiliser Consumption in the State during the Years 1996-97 to 1998-99

	1996-97	1997-98	1998-99
Fertiliser consumption in terms of Nutrients (N+P+K) in M.T.	795.79	946.65	977.54

Biofertilisers

The biofertiliser was introduced in the State just four years back. Various trainings/demonstration were conducted to popularise the use of biofertilisers in crop production programme. The experts from RBDC, Imphal have so far imparted 3 trainings to the Field Officers and Extension Workers in the Directorate of Agriculture, Kohima, which helped in enhancing the technical know-how about biofertilisers.

The trained field level officers on the other hand have imparted training to the farmers and demonstrated the use of biofertilisers. The farmers are encouraged and are using biofertilisers.

The consumption of biofertilisers in the State during the years 1995-96 to 1997-98 are given in Table 16.3.

Table 16.3: Consumption of Biofertilisers in the State during the Years 1995-96 to 1997-98

Sl.No.	Name of the Biofertiliser	Consumption (in kgs)		
		1995-96	1996-97	1997-98
1.	Azotobacter	2,000	2,000	2,000
2.	Rhizobium	2,000	2,300	1,800
3.	Phosphatika	1,500	700	800
4.	Bicomposting culture	—	1,000	1,300
	Total	4,500	5,000	5,300

The Government of India has sanctioned an amount of Rs. 20 lakh for setting up of Biofertiliser Production Unit. The equipments/glasswares have been procured and the biofertilisers production is likely to start from next year.

Biocompost

The Agriculture Department has taken up programme on improved method of compost making. The demonstrations and trainings were conducted on preparation of Biocompost using fungal culture throughout the state. The knowledge about the method of Biocomposting and its integrated use along with chemical fertilisers and biofertilisers were imparted to the farmers.

During the years 1995-96 to 1997-98 the number of compost pit dug for preparing biocompost are given below:

Year	Nos. of Compost Pits
1995-96	900 Nos.
1996-97	405 Nos.
1997-98	1,200 Nos.

17

FERTILISER USE IN FRUIT CROPS OF NORTH-EASTERN REGION OF INDIA

— K. Chuba Ao

Fruit crops are mostly perennial in nature and are heavy removers of plant nutrients from the soil. Therefore, the use of fertilisers is a must for production of good quality crop and high yields. A sound knowledge on balanced and optimum dose application avoiding indiscriminate application is a must while using fertilisers. Investments in recommended doses are fully justified only when the best varieties are planted to ensure that the plants being nourished have the potential of giving high return. Planting of good and suitable planting material is particularly crucial in the case of fruit plants because the same tree is to be fed, watered, looked after and becomes a source of income for several years.

Nutrient Management in Tree/Fruit Crops

- Fruit trees have a long pre-bearing period and requirement of nutrients vary with age of the plant.
- Generally, they have a deep root system and remain at the same place for years together which calls for regular monitoring of soil.
- Fruit crops have distinct and lengthy phases of vegetative and reproductive development.
- For fruit trees, manures are recommended in the pit before planting and in future application each year usually increasing quantities as the tree grows till bearing when these are stabilised.
- The first application of fertiliser is in the pit when the soil is being prepared to receive the plant. After planting, fertilisers are applied at increasing quantities as the tree grows and the dose is stabilised after 3-10 years depending on the fruit crop.

— The growing trees, fertiliser is usually given 30-100 cm away from the trunk in a basin, ring or trench. It is mixed thoroughly in the basin area or given 20-30 cm deep in a trench and mixed or covered with soil. Fertiliser application is followed by irrigation. Application of fertiliser close to the trunk is avoided because the feeding roots are not expected to be there. For example: In citrus plants, root activity/feeder root zone is at 10-25 cm depth and 120 cm radius from the trunk. In mango, 1.2-2.4 cm from the trunk and at 30, 60 and 90 cm depth with maximum root activity at 30 cm depth. In grapes, 30 m away from the trunk and 15 cm depth.

— Micro-nutrient recommendations include both soil as well as foliar applications though foliar application is preferred. For foliar application, some knowledge regarding nutrient composition of fertiliser and preparation of spray solution is required per hectare. Normally, the following concentrations are recommended for the given micro-nutrients (FAO Fertiliser and Plant Nutrition Bulletin No. 7, 1983):

Mg	:	1% $MgSO_4$
B	:	0.2—0.5% Soluble
Cu	:	0.025% (100 g Cu as $CuSO_4$)
Fe	:	1—3% $FeSO_4$
Mn	:	0.5—2% $MnSO_4$
Mo	:	01—0.3% Amm. Molybdate
Zn	:	0.5% $ZnSO_4$ + 0.25% Lime

These sprays are usually to be repeated 2 to 3 times or more at 7-10 days interval in order to bring the deficiency under complete control.

Method of Manuring and Fertilisation

Different recommendations have been made for the different fruit crops for manuring and fertilisations. Different methods of application have also been advocated. They are mentioned as follows:

Mango

A precise knowledge of rooting and root system is an essential pre-requisite for scientific application of manures and fertilisers. Studies conducted at ICAR indicated that feeding roots of a full grown mango plant are located between 1.2-2.4 m from the trunk (Singh, 1978). It was reported that most of the feeding roots were found at 30, 60 and 90 cm with maximum concentration at 30 cm depth. These observations suggested that for better absorption by the plants, manures and fertilisers application should be done within this area.

Apply the whole FYM, all P_2O_5, one-third N, half K_2O in January, one-third N + half P_2O_5 in April and one-third N in July after harvesting. According to age apply manures and fertilisers around the trunk followed by light hoeing and irrigation. Increase the doses in the subsequent years as recommended according to region or location.

Deficiency of micro-nutrient is usually not encountered although deficiencies of Fe, Mn, Zn, B and Cu have been observed.

Citrus

Citrus is a nutrient loving plant which play an important role for proper growth and development of citrus. In addition to macro-nutrients, it requires macro-nutrients like Zn, Cu, Mn, Fe, Mo etc. Deficiency of these elements causes serious disorders and eventually lead to decline of the orchard. For sustained production and proper maintenance of orchard, regular manuring and fertilisation should be done. For non-bearing tree, fertiliser should be applied around the trunk leaving 15-30 cm radius. In bearing trees, since the whole area becomes covered with roots, fertilisers may be applied by broadcasting from trunk to trunk leaving about 30 cm from the tree trunk.

Upto 5 years, apply fertilisers in 2 splits, half in February, half in September. After 5 years, apply all P_2O_5 + half N + half K_2O in February and rest N + K_2O in April. When there is deficiency in micro-nutrients, they are usually supplied through foliar sprays preferably in fair weather in the evening. The concentrations usually recommended are Copper Sulphate 0.2 per cent, Zinc Sulphate 0.4 per cent, Manganese Sulphate 0.1 per cent, Borax 0.5 per cent and slaked lime 0.3 per cent in water to correct the deficiencies of the same.

From the fertiliser trials conducted in 15 years old Khasi Mandarin Orchard situated in acid soils of northern slopes of Khasi Hills, Meghalaya reported that:

1. 300 g N, 250 g P and 300 g K/tree/year was best for economic yield.
2. Foliar application of 2 per cent Magnesium Sulphate, 0.1 per

cent Boric acid during the end of April increased fruit yield significantly (Ghosh *et al.*, 1981).

Banana

The nutrient requirement of banana is very high because banana takes up more nutrients per unit area than almost any other crop and the high fertilisation requirement of banana is mainly due to their rapid and vigorous growth and high fruit yield.

Nitrogen should be applied in small doses at short intervals while Phosphorus (P) is applied at planting and Potash (K) in 2 split doses—one at planting and another at the time of initiation of flowers. Summerville (1944) reported that:

1. Nutrients should be plentily available at the time of planting and initiation of ratoons.
2. Potash applied in the first two months has a greater influence on the number of hands produced than when applied after shooting.
3. The uptake of phosphorus is more rapid when the plants are 2-3 months old.

The beneficial effects of micro-nutrients such as Mg, Fe, Mn, B, Cu, Mo, Zn on the growth and yield of banana have been reported by many investigators.

Grapes

The fertiliser requirement of a grapevine is influenced by many factors like soil fertility status, age and vigour, yield potentiality, climate, vine management etc. Therefore, recommendations made for one region may not hold good for another region.

The active feeding roots are found in the range from 30-40 cm depth. At the initial stage, the grapevine mainly take nutrients initially applied for filling the pits. Whatever manures and fertilisers required are applied 30 cm away from the plant in the circular ring in the first year and in the subsequent years, these are applied in 15 cm depth furrow made around the vines (root area of the vines). Micro-nutrients of 0.2 per cent Boric acid, 0.05 per cent Iron, 0.5 per cent Mn, 0.2 per cent Zn in the form of foliar spray have been found to be beneficial for growth and production.

Litchi

Litchi is very responsive to environment conditions which influence the vegetative, flowering and fruiting cycle of the plant. The young litchi plants are sensitive to fertiliser burn, therefore, the suggested fertiliser recommended are applied 20 cm beyond the trunk.

Apply all phosphorus, one-third Nitrogen and half Potash in January, one-third N + half Potash in April and one-third N in July after harvesting. According to age, apply fertilisers under the tree canopy leaving 60-90 cm around the trunk, give light hoeing followed by irrigation. The fertiliser rate depends on the tree size, vigour, crop load, cultivar, spacing, climate and soil type.

Table 17.1: N, P and K Doses for Well-grown Litchi Trees

Tree Age (years)	Canopy Diameter (m)	N (g/tree)	P_2O_5 (g/tree)	K_2O (g/tree)
4—5	1.0—1.5	200	80	300
6—7	2.0—2.5	300	100	450
8—9	3.0—3.5	400	130	550
10—11	4.0—4.5	500	170	700
12—13	5.0—5.5	600	200	800
14—15	6.0—6.5	800	250	1,200
> 15	6.5	1,000	300	1,400

Source: Menzel and Simpson (1986d).

Pineapple

Pineapple requires abundant supply of nitrogen and potash than phosphorus. Increased yield and improvement in quality of pineapple by application of fertilisers have been reported.

Apply all FYM in the last ploughing, all P + K + half N as band or line placement. Apply half N as foliar spray in 6 parts every 2 months. Dissolve 450 g Urea in 10 litres of water and spray in 200 plants. Soil application of Mg (0.64/pl), Boron (0.24/pl), Fe (0.64 g/pl) hastened flowering and increased yield.

Application of fertilisers in two split doses, once the onset of monsoon (May-June) and again at the end of rainy season (September-October) after the fruits are harvested has also been recommended for growth and yield. Fertilisation is followed by earthing around the stem.

Table 17.2: Area and Production of Fruits in North East India (1986-87)

State/Territory	Area ('000 ha)	Proportionate Share %	Production ('000 tonnes)	Proportionate Share %	Productivity (tonnes/ha)
Arunachal Pradesh	9.62	0.33	22.33	0.08	2.32
Assam	41.58	1.41	550.74	2.08	13.25
Manipur	17.03	0.58	175.26	0.66	10.29
Meghalaya	25.98	0.88	175.61	0.66	6.76
Mizoram	33.82	1.15	18.94	0.07	0.56
Nagaland	3.24	0.11	5.88	0.02	1.81
Sikkim	9.38	0.32	2.73	0.01	0.29
Tripura	34.73	1.18	277.72	1.05	8.00
India	2,940.33	100.00	26,512.68	100.00	9.02

Source: Eighth Plan Working Group for Horticulture and Plantation Crops.

Guava

Apply all FYM + half NPK in March-April and rest NPK in September-October in shallow according to spread of the tree canopy. To correct Zn deficiency, spray 55 g Zinc Sulphate + 85 g slaked lime in 100 litres of water or 100-300 g Zinc Sulphate/plant in the soil. Irrigation should be done after fertiliser application.

Papaya

The nutrition of papaya differs from other fruit crops because of its quick growth, continuous fruiting habit and heavy fruit yield.

Apply NPK in 6 splits doses every two months by mixing in soil followed by irrigation. Manure mixture of 40 kg FYM + 2 kg SSP in 225 litres of water, keep in covered for 3 days, mix and add water to make 450 litres and applied @ half litre per plant every two weeks followed by irrigation.

Apple, Pear, Peach, Plum

Apply P and K in December, half N in February-March three weeks before flowering and rest in March-April just after fruit set. For apple, to overcome mineral deficiency, apply 1 per cent urea + 0.3 per cent Agromine or 0.25 per cent Multiplex at 15-20 days intervals.

Table 17.3: Nutrient Removal by Some Crops (kg/ha)

Crop	Yields (t/ha)	N	P_2O_5	K_2O	MgO	S
Apple	25	100	45	180	40	n.n
Banana	40	250	60	1,000	140	15
Citrus	30	100	60	350	40	30
Grape	20	170	60	200	60	30
Mango	15	100	25	100	75	n.n
Papaya	50	90	25	130	15	10
Pineapple	50	185	55	350	110	20

Note: Average values taken from various sources as summarised by Kemmler, G. and Hobt, H. in "Potassium—A Product of Nature", Kali-und-Salz AG, F.R. Germany.

Assam

Table 17.4: Fertiliser Doses in Assam

Crop	Space etc.	Age. etc.	N	P_2O_5	K_2O	FYM etc.
Fruits						
Pineapple	44,000/ha		12	2	12 g/plant	15 t/ha
Banana	1.8 × 2.4 m		110	35	330 g/plant	12 kg/plant
Papaya	1.8 × 1.8 m		110	50	100 g/tree	
Jackfruit	10-12 m	bearing	210	160	1,000 g/tree	20-30 kg/tree
Guava	5-7 m	bearing	630	320	1,200 g/tree	20 kg/tree
Litchi	9-12 m	bearing	60	40	60 g/tree	
Sapota	7-9 m	bearing	See text below			20-25 kg/tree
Mango	12 × 12 m	1 yr old	0	400	500 g/tree	10 kg/tree
		bearing	420	400	1,250 g/tree	100 kg/tree
Assam lemon	3 × 3 m	1 yr old	150	100	150 g/tree	5 kg/tree
		4 yr old	600	400	600 g/tree	20 kg/tree
Mandarin orange	5 × 5 m	2nd yr	150	120	100 g/tree	
		3rd yr	300	240	200 g/tree	
		6th yr	750	600	500 g/tree	
		7th & above	750	600	500 g/tree	

Arunachal Pradesh

Table 17.5: Fertiliser Doses in Arunachal Pradesh

Crop	Plants/ha	Age etc.	N	P_2O_5	K_2O	FYM etc.
(1)	(2)	(3)	(4)	(5)	(6)	(7)
Fruits						
Apple	400	1st yr	50	30	30 g/tree	20 kg/tree
Pear	400	2nd yr	100	60	60 g/tree	25 kg/tree

(Contd.)

Table 17.5: (*Contd.*)

(1)	(2)	(3)	(4)	(5)	(6)	(7)
Plum	400	3rd yr	150	90	90 g/tree	30 kg/tree
Peach	278	4th yr	200	120	120 g/tree	35 kg/tree
Almond	278	5th yr	250	150	150 g/tree	40 kg/tree
Apricot	278	6th yr	300	180	180 g/tree	45 kg/tree
		7th yr	350	170	210 g/tree	50 kg/tree
Lemon	400	1st yr	90	90	90 g/tree	20 kg/tree
		2nd yr	150	150	200 g/tree	25 kg/tree
		3rd yr	200	200	300 g/tree	30 kg/tree
Mandarin	494	4th yr	250	250	500 g/tree	35 kg/tree
Sweet orange	278	5th yr	350	350	600 g/tree	40 kg/tree
		6th yr	400	400	700 g/tree	45 kg/tree
		7th yr	450	450	900 g/tree	50 kg/tree
Pineapple	13,333		30	20	20 g/pl	2 kg/tree
Banana (dwarf)	2,500		180	100	225 kg/ha	20 kg/tree
Banana (tall)	625					
Papaya	525		40	75	75 kg/ha	30 t/ha
Guava	278		50	80	100 kg/ha	20 t/ha
Litchi	400		40	70	90 kg/ha	20 t/ha
Pomegranate	625		40	70	90 kg/ha	

Mizoram

Table 17.6: Fertiliser Doses in Mizoram

Crop	Spacing	Age etc.	N	P_2O_5	K_2O	FYM etc.
Fruits						
Orange & other Citrus fruits	3-5 m	2nd yr	150	120	100 g/tree	10-15 kg/tree
		3rd yr	300	240	200 g/tree	10-15 kg/tree
		4th yr	450	350	300 g/tree	10-15 kg/tree
		7th & above	900	720	600 g/tree	10-15 kg/tree
Pineapple	44,000/ha		10	15	10 g/plant	10-15 t/ha
Banana	2 × 2 m		100	50	300 g/plant	10-20 kg
Papaya	1.8 × 1.8 m		150	300	200 g/plant	10-20 kg

Source: Directorate of Agriculture, Aizawl, Mizoram.

Conclusion

The requirement of fruits is increasing day by day to meet the demands of the ever-increasing population and since there is no possibility to increase the cultivable land. The only possibility to meet the requirement is to increase the production through application of fertilisers and manures in the right doses and methods.

REFERENCES

Singh, R.N. (1978)."Nutrition", In: *Mango Low-Priced Book*, Series No. 3, ICAR, New Delhi, p. 66-73.

Ghosh, S.P.; Verma, A.N. and Sheo Govind (1981). "Nutritional Requirement of Khasi Mandarin Orange (*C. reticulata Blanco*) for Higher Yields in Meghalaya", *Nat. Symp. Trop. & Sub Trop. Fruit Crops*, Bangalore, Abstr., pp. 48.

Summerville, W.A.T. (1944). "Studies in Nutrition as Qualified by Development", In: *Musa Cavendishi, Queensland J. Agri. Sci*, 1: 1-127.

Menzel, C.M. and Simpson, D.R. (1986d). *Proc. Ist Nat. lychee Sem.*, Australia, pp. 22-36.

INDEX